DR. SCHUBINER IS A COMPASSIONATE AND DEVOTED PHYSICIAN whose unique approach has helped hundreds of people—including many of my own patients—heal their pain and reclaim their lives. This book will give thousands more access to this revolutionary program.

> —*Michael C. Hsu, MD, Physical Medicine and Musculoskeletal Specialist, Kaiser-Northwest Permanente, Portland, Oregon*

HOWARD SCHUBINER'S WORK is a tremendous advancement in the field of pain relief. His visionary thinking and comprehensive program will heal untold numbers of chronic pain patients. The book should be required reading for all patients and physicians who deal with chronic pain.

> —*John Stracks, MD, Department of Family Medicine, Integrative Medicine Program, Northwestern University, Chicago, Illinois*

UNLEARN YOUR PAIN EXPLAINS THE SCIENCE behind chronic pain in a common sense way that everyone will understand. Dr. Schubiner's revolutionary program is based upon his groundbreaking research and really works. This book is the answer to your long search for the cure to your pain.

> —*Steven Gurgevich, Ph.D., Clinical Assistant Professor of Medicine, Arizona Center for Integrative Medicine, University of Arizona College of Medicine*

I WAS A FIBROMYALGIA SUFFERER for over twenty-five years, and despite excellent medical care, my severe pain persisted. Dr. Schubiner's program helped me uncover the root causes of my pain and gave me the tools to deal with it. *Unlearn Your Pain* is a truly astounding program. Within the first week, I could not believe how much the pain decreased and my energy levels increased. I continue to be pain free because *Unlearn Your Pain* is now my recipe for living.
  —*Fran Baiamonte, Burlington, Connecticut*

I WAS DIAGNOSED WITH TWO HERNIATED DISCS and a pinched nerve as a result of my auto accident. I tried every medical treatment from physical therapy to injections to heavy narcotics. The cycle of pain and suffering continued for three-and-a-half years. It wasn't until I took Dr. Schubiner's Mind Body program that my pain subsided.
  —*Marnina Sullivan, Detroit, Michigan*

AFTER SUFFERING WITH SEVERE HAND PAIN for more than three years and not getting any relief from more than eight doctors plus several alternative healers, I had begun to lose hope of ever recovering. Dr. Schubiner's program explained my pain in a way that made perfect sense, and after completing the program, I can honestly say that my pain is virtually gone. In addition, I now understand myself much better, and this has made me a better person.
  —*Edward Samuels, Chicago, Illinois*

AT A TIME WHEN I THOUGHT I WAS OUT OF OPTIONS to deal with severe bladder and pelvic pain, Dr. Schubiner's program gave me the tools to take control of my life and manage my symptoms. All other traditional treatments had failed. I am forever grateful, and I continue to employ these techniques in many aspects of my life.
  —*Erica El-Alayli, Brighton, Michigan*

AFTER SEVEN YEARS OF SEVERE BACK PAIN which no doctor, drugs, physiotherapist, chiropractor, acupuncturist, or massage therapist could fix, this program gave me relief within a couple of months. The techniques are easy to use, have given me great insight, and, best of all, relieved my pain. I recommend it highly — it changed my life!
  —*Lisa Manchester, London, UK*

DR. SCHUBINER'S PROGRAM NOT ONLY HELPED ME break a cycle of nearly continuous headache, it provided me with a broader, deeper, and very useful understanding of how psychological and emotional issues impact my physical well-being.
  —*Eric Keller, Ferndale, Michigan*

I HAVE SUFFERED FROM PAIN since I was a teenager. I have been diagnosed with more disorders than I could name. But no one was ever sure what was really wrong. Dr. Schubiner's course saved my life. Thank God I now realize that I have Mind Body Syndrome.
    —*Walter Lanier, Anderson, South Carolina*

PHYSICAL THERAPY, CORTISONE INJECTIONS, and chiropractic treatment didn't help the intense pain in my back and down my leg. Over a year, I spent thousands of dollars without relief. Three weeks after I started Dr. Schubiner's program, the pain was gone. I am still amazed that it worked, and I cannot be more grateful.
    —*Gwen Clark, New Baltimore, Michigan*

THIS PROGRAM TAUGHT ME that my life experiences had caused my pain. The exercises brought about incredible insights, and the words flowed out of my head and onto the paper. A huge weight had been lifted, and consequently my back pain is gone.
    —*Denise Marsh, Royal Oak, Michigan*

AS A HEALTH CARE PROVIDER, I was skeptical when I heard about Mind Body Syndrome. Thanks to Dr. Schubiner, I now understand the connection between my emotional state and my physical pain. His program gave me techniques that I have used to control my symptoms and reclaim my life. Thank you so much, Dr. Schubiner.
    —*Diane Olsem, RN, Brighton Township, Michigan*

DR. SCHUBINER'S MIND BODY SYNDROME PROGRAM enabled me to free myself from fibromyalgia pain which was basically running my life for thirteen years. I am finally on the road to recovery and feel so much more in control of my life and my health.
    —*Cindy Corey, Livonia, Michigan*

I USED DR. SCHUBINER'S COURSE after everything else failed to stop chronic hamstring pain. His course told me exactly what to do and what not to do, on a daily basis. It took me about two months, but I am now able to walk, work out at the gym, and I now don't worry about my every move.
    —*Steve Hansen, Easton, Maryland*

DR. SCHUBINER'S MIND BODY PROGRAM TAUGHT ME that I have control over my back pain. I quit worrying about all the "physical" problems that I had been told were wrong with my neck and back and started to concentrate on what was going on in my mind. When I realized how much pain had become my identity, I began to heal. Where I could only see a lifetime of pain, I have now regained a healthy and active life.
    —*Cathy Gibson, Northville, Michigan*

unlearn your pain

Notes on the meditations for your book page

THERE ARE SEVERAL AUDIO GUIDED MEDITATIONS designed to go along with this program. They are used for both of the books, *Unlearn Your Pain* and *Unlearn Your Anxiety and Depression*.

You can access these meditations by going to my website, unlearnyourpain.com and clicking on the Meditations pull down menu at the top of the home page. The password is: meditations

You will come to a page with the meditations, which you can play from the website or download to Windows Media Player or iTunes.

If you would like to stay abreast of news, blogposts and training opportunities, you can receive emails by sending me an email at hschubiner@gmail.com asking to be placed on our mailing list.

To your health,
Howard Schubiner, MD
hschubiner@gmail.com

Copyright, fourth edition © 2022
by Mind Body Publishing, Pleasant Ridge, MI

All rights reserved
Printer: Sheridan Books, Inc.
CD Replication: Kopy-Rite
Printed in the United States of America
Cover Photograph: Getty Images, Photodisc
Author Photograph: Rob Vinson
Design and Layout: Eric Keller
Set in Trade Gothic and ITC Century.

Schubiner, Howard with Betzold, Michael
Unlearn Your Pain: a 28-day process to reprogram your brain
ISBN: 979-8-9864716-0-0 (fourth edition)

Howard Schubiner, MD
www.unlearnyourpain.com

unlearn your pain

A 28-DAY PROCESS
TO REPROGRAM YOUR BRAIN

By Howard Schubiner, MD,
with Michael Betzold

FOURTH EDITION

MIND ✳ BODY
PUBLISHING

To my wonderful parents, Lorraine and Elliot I. Schubiner

May you have the commitment
To heal what has hurt you,
To allow it to come close to you,
And, in the end, become one with you.
— Gaelic blessing

DISCLAIMER: Reading this book does not establish a doctor-patient relationship with Dr. Schubiner, nor does it offer diagnosis and/or treatment for medical conditions. You should consult with your own doctors to make sure that your condition does not require medical intervention and that an approach that includes a consideration of the role that the mind plays in your symptoms is acceptable. You should also make sure that your doctor approves of any change in activities that you might undertake.

This book does not offer specific recommendations about the use of medications or about changing your use of medications. You should decide along with your physician if you should alter or stop any of your medications. In particular, stopping certain medications can cause physical or psychological symptoms if the process is not done carefully. The program suggests that you review stressful events in your life and asks you to view them in relation to how you are feeling, physically and psychologically. If you are in counseling, you should consult with your therapist or counselor to make sure that they think you can participate in this program. If you develop emotional difficulties during the course of taking this program, it is critical that you consult with your physician or therapist. Many people have found that it is helpful (and sometimes necessary) to use this program with the aid of a counselor or therapist.

table of contents

Notes on *Unlearn Your Pain* and *Unlearn Your Anxiety and Depression*

In 2014, I published *Unlearn Your Anxiety and Depression.* It takes a critical look at the current medical understanding and treatment of these disorders and suggests an alternative model, a mind body point of view. As I have accumulated experience in treating individuals with anxiety, depression and chronic pain, I have come to the conclusion that the mind body approach as outlined in *Unlearn Your Pain* is an effective treatment model for most patients with these disorders. With the publication of the third edition of *Unlearn Your Pain*, I have decided to update the workbook section to make it applicable to anxiety and depression, along with other mind body disorders.

Both *Unlearn Your Pain* and *Unlearn Your Anxiety and Depression.* are available in print and eBook formats. There are also eBook versions of each book including just the first five chapters without the self-guided recovery program/workbook. The workbook sections of the books are identical. See unlearnyourpain.com for more information.

How to Use This Book

If your first thought at seeing this book is that it's just too big, you wouldn't be the first person to think that and you would also be correct. It is too big. It can appear overwhelming, in fact. It is filled with information about the mind-body connection, with exercises to complete in writing and in your imagination, and with specific techniques for rewiring your brain, and much more. Many people never start it or get upset with some of the ideas in it.

However, you're picking this book up for a reason. There is something not right in your body. And maybe there are some things that need to be changed in your mind too and even in your life as well. This book will help you figure it out, I promise. It may take some time and it will take some effort. But I can tell you it will be worth it.

Take this book as an opportunity to explore what is going on in your body and in your mind and in your life. Take it slowly, little by little, so that you can really understand what I'm saying and so that you can evaluate if this material applies to you. I would guess that much of the information here will apply to you, but I also guess that not all of it will apply to you. Don't worry about that. If some of the material here seems off-putting to you or not relevant to your situation, that's fine. I expect that to happen. But don't "throw the baby out with the bath water." Please be open to these ideas. Look carefully for what applies to you and you will find ways to recover. Feel free to ignore parts that do not apply to you, but don't let those parts get in the way of the things that will be useful, in fact, essential to you. Think of this book as a toolbox that you can use and find the tools that you need. Many people have recovered from chronic pain and other associated conditions by just reading and understanding this material. Some spend a lot of time doing the writing exercises, while others do little or no writing at all. Some investigate stressful life experiences and traumatic events using emotional awareness and expression therapy, while others avoid these issues and this work. You will chart your own path as you go through this book. It will be worth your time and effort.

Howard Schubiner, MD

August, 2022

preface

My mentor in medical school was Dr. Muir Clapper, a very wise and aging physician, who knew that I was the kind of person who wanted to challenge the status quo. He told me, "Howard, get your tickets." He meant that, if I wanted to shake things up in medicine, I should get good training to develop the expertise I would need. I listened to his advice.

Since I graduated from medical school in 1978, I have become board certified in Internal Medicine, Pediatrics, and Adolescent Medicine. I spent half of my career at Wayne State University Medical School in Detroit and became a full Professor there in 2002. I have conducted research studies, taught medical students and residents, authored articles in medical journals, and practiced medicine for thirty-eight years. I participated in the creation of a holistic medical center, and I studied acupuncture in China. I have also been listed on the Best Doctors in America list on several occasions. I got my tickets, but what was I to do with them?

A good friend from medical school, Dr. Ernie Yoder, offered me a position at Providence Hospital (now Ascension Providence Hospital) in 2002 and I asked him what they wanted me to do there. He replied, "Well, what do you want to do?" After much soul-searching, I accepted. Within a year, Ernie told me about a patient of his who had a remarkable recovery from severe back and hip pain. He suggested that I take a look at the book that helped her become pain free within a few weeks. She had read *The Mindbody Prescription* by Dr. John Sarno, a rehabilitation physician at New York University. Almost forty years ago, Dr. Sarno realized that pain was a relatively common manifestation of stress and emotional reactions to stress. He became a pioneer in the field of mind body medicine and has helped innumerable people through his work and his writing. Yet only a relatively small number of physicians have incorporated this work into their practices. In fact, few physicians are even aware that syndromes such as back and neck pain, headaches, fatigue, fibromyalgia, temporomandibular joint syndrome, and bladder syndromes can be caused by stress and neural circuits in the brain that are very real, yet occur in the absence of tissue damage.

When I looked back on my own life, I realized that I too had experienced physical symptoms in response to stress and emotions. My neck began to hurt in 1983 and has caused me significant disability over the years. I've had headaches, diarrhea, leg pain and back pain from time to time as well. Now that I am fully aware of the incredible connection between the mind and the body, I am almost always able to get rid of the aches and pains that arise by recognizing them for what they are: physical symptoms as a manifestation of stress, worry, anxiety, fears, anger, and the many other emotions that come with being human.

In 2003, I started the Mind Body Medicine program at Providence Hospital in Southfield, Michigan. I have worked extremely hard to find innovative exercises and approaches to help my patients. I have also learned a tremendous amount from my patients. They have shown great courage in the face of severe pain and adversity, and they have helped me to expand the program and make it better.

Two significant things usually occur in people who enter the Mind Body Medicine program. First, their physical symptoms improve. This is the case for the majority of patients within the first month of taking the program. Many others improve later, though not all patients have gotten rid of all of their symptoms. The second thing that typically occurs is that most people learn to understand themselves much better. They learn what issues in their life have the greatest impact on them and why. They begin to see that issues from their childhood often influence their response to issues occurring in the present. And most importantly, they learn techniques for dealing with the issues most relevant to them in both the past and present. In short, they begin to achieve mastery and a sense of control over their emotions, their reactions to stress, and most importantly, their own bodies. I have found that even those people whose physical symptoms do not improve fully, or as much as they would like, are still grateful for the program because it helps them learn so much about themselves.

Because of these gratifying results in my work, I have decided to write this book so more people can have access to the program that my patients have found so beneficial. I am also writing this book to educate physicians about Mind Body Syndrome. Modern medicine has made many advances for heart disease and cancer. However, for the millions of people with Mind Body Syndrome, medical interventions have not been helpful and are actually a part of the problem. To really help people with these syndromes, we need to change medicine by educating both the public and physicians to recognize and treat these disorders more effectively, which can eliminate a great deal of needless suffering.

To your health,
Howard Schubiner, MD
Southfield, Michigan
August 2022

acknowledgments

I am fortunate to have many people to thank. I wanted to write this book for a few years but did not start because the task seemed too overwhelming to undertake on top of my other responsibilities. My good friend, Michael Betzold, an excellent writer, gave me both the encouragement and the resources (his fine writing and editing skills) to complete this project. Another friend, Maureen Dunphy, who designed the course "Journaling as Writing Tool" at Oakland University, provided me with resources about and contributed the initial design of several writing exercises.

I wouldn't have known about the underlying cause of chronic pain without an interaction with a longtime friend, colleague, and former supervisor, Dr. Ernest Yoder. Ernie set me on this course with a single conversation and then allowed me to develop a new line of practice and research within our hospital. Dr. John Sarno is a pioneer and visionary who had the insight and courage to find a new way to understand back pain almost fifty years ago. I hope that I can help to expand upon his work and bring it into the mainstream of medical practice.

The work of several scientists and authors has been extremely influential, and I'd like to thank them for their cutting-edge work. Drs. Daniel Wegner, Timothy D. Wilson, and Joseph LeDoux wrote books that opened my mind to some of the science behind Mind Body Syndrome (see Appendix). This work has been dramatically advanced by understanding that the brain works by a process called, predictive processing. I have learned a great deal about this by reading the works of Lisa Feldman Barrett, Andy Clark and Karl Friston and others. This also reflects these revolutionary concepts that have taken this work to a new level. My mindfulness meditation teachers, Jon Kabat-Zinn, Saki Santorelli, Melissa Blacker, Ferris Urbanowski, and Elana Rosenbaum, taught me the skills that have helped me infuse this program with the thought and practices of mindfulness. This book has been influenced by the work of two pioneers in psychotherapy, Drs. Habib Davanloo and Allan Abbass. I believe that their work is underappreciated in modern psychiatry and psychology and can be of great benefit in the healing process that allows the body to rid itself of pain and other symptoms.

Finally, I wholeheartedly thank my colleagues in the newly founded Psychophysiologic Disorders Association, including David Clarke, David Schechter, David Hanscom, Jessica Shahinian, Jessican Oifer and others. They are also pioneers working to inform the public and the wider medical community about these disorders.

I have been fortunate to be able to work with several excellent researchers and thinkers, such as Drs. Dan Clauw and Dave Williams from the University of Michigan. Dr. Michael Hsu worked tirelessly with me on the fibromyalgia research study and helped me sharpen my concepts. Dr. John Stracks has been a great source of support and the co-organizer of our first Mind Body professional meeting.

I am indebted to Alan Gordon, Yoni Ashar and Christie Uipi as amazing colleagues in further developing and studying these ideas. They contributed brilliant ideas and worked tirelessly on the Boulder back pain study that has showed the value of Pain Reprocessing Therapy as a powerful treatment for mind-body syndromes. Michael Doninno has also contributed greatly to studying this work. Mark Lumley at Wayne State University has worked with me on all of the studies and has contributed his massive knowledge base, critical thinking and tremendous efforts to furthering this work. He and I developed Emotional Awareness and Expression Therapy as a method of addressing unprocessed emotions and stressful life events, upon which much of this book relies. I would also like to thank Kent Bassett and Marion Cunningham for their heroic efforts in directing and producing the documentary, This Might Hurt, which has illuminated this work in poignant, accessible and powerful ways. There are three talented practitioners and teachers who have allowed me to team up with them in developing training opportunities for medical professionals and others to spread these ideas: Alicia Batson (on OVID Dx, a mobile training app), Hal Greenham (Freedom From Chronic Pain) and Charlie Merrill (Beyond Pain Education).

I would like to express my gratitude to Eric Keller and Rob Vinson, who are not only good friends but very talented in their fields of graphic design and photography/videography, respectively. I thank one of my oldest friends, Mike Blumenthal, who is now also my website designer and advisor. I am very grateful to my daughter, Lindsay, for her editing skills and to my brother-in-law and good friend, George Nolte, for his expert proofreading. And I acknowledge my men's group, the intrepid Council of Men, who have supported and challenged me for over thirty years.

The people who seek my help and entrust their lives and their stories to me are the reason I keep doing this work. (The names of several patients in this book have been altered to protect their identities.) They are inspirational in their courage to stand up for themselves and, often, to the medical profession. It has taken me forty years of being a doctor to begin to understand the concepts and ideas contained in the book. Very few of these ideas are actually original though. I have worked hard to understand them and learned from people much smarter than me. In fact, much of what I have learned has come from the patients I have seen and the people who write to me asking for help. They are the people who helped me write this book. They are people just like you, who just desperately need to feel better. They teach me new things every day about the mind and the body, and they help me to be a better doctor and person.

People often look at me and think "This guy's kind of old, when is he going to retire?" Yet, I can't think of a better job: helping people recover from symptoms that they are often told are incurable, teaching other medical professionals how to do this work, honoring the work of giants in medicine and science who have inspired me, helping people see who they really are and what they need to do to thrive, challenging old dogmas and getting both accolades and ire, which keeps me always questioning and learning.

I thank my children, Lindsay and Gabe, who have taught me many things and who give my life great meaning. My parents have given me incredible love and support every day of my life, and I owe everything to them. Finally, my wife and best friend of forty-five years, Val Overholt, allows me to think I'm brilliant and laughs at my foibles. On a daily basis, she provides me with what one of my wise ancestors suggested is necessary to be content and balanced: keeping a piece of paper in one pocket which reads, "For my sake the world was created," and in the other pocket, "I am but dust and ashes."

chapter 1
The Truth About Your Pain

Telling people about Mind Body Syndrome is like telling them
that the earth is round, when they KNOW that it's flat!
— Anonymous patient

Vitiant artus aegrae contagia mentis.
(When the mind is ill at ease, the body is affected.) — Ovid

It hurts.

Your pain is awful. Your misery is unrelenting. No matter what you do, you can't get rid of it.

You went to your doctor, and he told you that you had a medical condition: degenerative disc disease, spinal stenosis, fibromyalgia, irritable bowel syndrome, whiplash, or something else. Your doctor prescribed drugs. You took them, but they didn't really help. Maybe you had injections or you even had surgery, but that didn't stop the pain, whether it was in your back, your head, your neck, your gut, or all over.

Perhaps you have explored alternative medicine. Maybe you took herbal remedies, had therapeutic massages, or saw a chiropractor. You're considering acupuncture, hypnosis, and even crystals, if that might help. Some of these treatments may have provided temporary or partial relief, but still the pain is there, day after day after day. You might have seen alternative health practitioners who gave you different diagnoses, gave you supplements or herbs, or changed your diet. You've gone to so many health practitioners that you are starting to feel no one can help you because no one understands the real problem. Maybe your doctor even referred you to a psychiatrist or psychologist, suggesting that your pain isn't real—that it's all in your head.

But you know you're not imagining your pain. You're not faking it to gain attention or sympathy. It's about time someone in the medical profession recognized that the pain in your body is real. It's about time that someone in the medical profession told you that there is a reason for your pain and a way to cure it.

I am that doctor, and I'm telling you: Your pain is real, there is a reason for it, and there is a cure for it. The only way to relieve the pain is to find the underlying cause of it, to get to the bottom of it. The problem is not in your head. It's in your diagnosis.

Some doctors may say you have a serious medical condition, but if they don't know how to cure it, their diagnosis doesn't help you. Perhaps alternative health practitioners will tell you that your spine is not properly aligned or your aura is out of whack or your chi is diminished. All of these are different ways of looking at your body, but none of them will succeed if they're not correctly diagnosing why your body hurts.

I have some good news for you. Unless you have a medical problem resulting in clear pathology in your body (which can be determined by routine medical tests), your pain can be cured. Following this program, you can take some relatively easy steps to vanquish it.

Like tens of millions of Americans and countless others around the globe who suffer from chronic back pain, muscle pain, headaches, migraines, stomach pain, and other misdiagnosed conditions, you're hurting because of overly sensitized neural circuits in the brain. These connections have created a vicious cycle of pain that can last for months, years, or even decades unless you do what it takes to stop it. This cycle of pain signals has been "learned" by your brain—and the longer these signals keep firing, the more sensitized and overactive the neural circuits become, and the more pain you feel.

The event that started this horrible pain cycle could have been an injury or a stressful event in your life, or it could have come out of the blue. A very careful and detailed look at your current situation and your life history will reveal how your brain is actually creating this pain and perpetuating the vicious cycle. As I will explain in detail, our brains create the pain that we feel, whether that pain is caused by a serious injury or by stress. Most people and most doctors are not aware of this fact. And, most importantly, since our brains generate pain, all pain is the same, all pain comes from the brain, all pain is real.

The best news is that you don't have to live the rest of your life with this pain. Whether you've had it for a few weeks or for many years, it can be beaten. Just as your brain has learned to make your body hurt, you can use your brain to unlearn the pain. There's a way to retrain your brain so that your body isn't contorted into pain. This book will explain how this can be done without drugs or surgery, by anyone with the motivation to do so.

In fact, if you begin to understand this syndrome and recognize what causes it, you've already taken a powerful first step. And the rest of the steps, though they require wholehearted commitment, are not difficult. They are all explained in this book, and the whole program is laid out for you to work through. Improvement may occur within days or weeks, even if you've been suffering for a long time. And by doing the program you can get more than temporary or partial relief. You can achieve complete freedom from the pain and distress that have hobbled you.

Starting today, you can break the vicious cycle of pain. And you can start to use your mental energy to overcome your limitations and rebuild your life.

I know this is true because I have done it myself. I've changed my understanding of the source of my pain, and I now can identify when the stresses of everyday life produce pain in my body and I can overcome them.

More importantly, I've seen the same transformation in hundreds of my patients.

This program is not risky or far out. It doesn't require belief in an alternative paradigm of medicine or philosophy. The work of unlearning your pain is based on solid science and common sense.

The Neural Circuits of Pain

Pain begins when circuits from the brain are stimulated or "fired." Over time, these circuits can become "wired" into the brain's circuitry. The brain learns this chronic pain, even though there is no serious medical condition in the body, and even though any injury that may have precipitated the pain has long ago healed.

Everyone knows that if you break your arm, it will hurt, but after the fracture heals in a few weeks, the pain will disappear. But I have seen hundreds of people whose pain began with an injury but lasted five, ten, even twenty years. Why? The body has surely healed. The answer to this puzzle is found in the neural circuits in the brain.

Many people have heard about "phantom limb" pain, the pain that is felt in the area of an arm or a leg that has been amputated. There is clearly nothing wrong with that area—it isn't even there—yet this pain can be severe. We now know that this pain is caused by the creation of neural circuits in the brain.

The good news is that the brain can be retrained to get out of ruts that produce pain and to activate the normal, non-pain circuits that are waiting to be used. An increasing body of evidence is showing that the brain has amazing neuroplasticity—it is always learning and creating new neural circuits. All you have to do is tap into that power and use it to reprogram your response to pain and to the factors that intensify that pain.

There are three major components of the nervous system that create the vicious cycle of pain: the nerves that send pain signals from the body to the brain; the brain itself, where those nerve signals are interpreted; and the nerves that send signals back to the body. The best way to end chronic pain and other chronic symptoms is by retraining the brain, the controller of the nervous system. Most people don't realize that the brain can both create and cure chronic painful conditions. Unfortunately, there are few doctors who understand this simple fact. Doctors who don't know that learned neural circuits can cause real, physical pain believe that all pain originates from some kind of tissue damage in the body. When they cannot identify the tissue damage, they are perplexed and sometimes blame the patient or doubt that there is real pain. Modern medicine's treatment for chronic pain usually consists of pain medications, injections or surgery. While these may help to some degree by controlling symptoms, they don't get to the root cause of the pain and therefore cannot reverse it. For people with pain caused by learned neural circuits, cutting-edge brain research demonstrates that it is possible to change these circuits and interrupt this vicious cycle.

Stress and Pain

Pain cannot be felt without the brain, which interprets tissue damage signals and can transform them into the experience of pain. Of course, it is important to be able to feel pain so we can protect ourselves from danger. However, these circuits often tend to get reinforced over time by our reactions to the pain. Just about everyone who has chronic pain will react to that pain with fear, anger, anxiety, frustration, and other worrisome thoughts and emotions. These thoughts and emotions trigger increased pain by an "amplification" process in the brain.

Thoughts and emotions, whether we are aware of them or whether they are subconscious, are major factors in producing chronic pain and related syndromes. In addition, the stress that frequently accompanies these symptoms, such as decreased activity, decreased income, and more difficult relationships, adds to the problem by making the stress-producing neural circuits stronger.

In this kind of situation, your brain will continue to produce pain because that's the only way your brain knows how to deal with these stresses. The truth is that your mind can twist your body into a cycle of very real pain.

It is common for people with difficult emotional experiences in their childhood or their recent past to have this same amplification of pain. In fact, certain traumatic experiences in childhood leave an imprint on the brain, making it more likely to develop the vicious pain cycle. People who have a great deal of unresolved stress are also more likely to have chronic pain. Almost everyone has stress to some degree, and in many people it results, sooner or later, in chronic pain that can range from mild and intermittent to intense and unrelenting. And there are many symptoms in addition to pain that can be caused by these wayward connections, such as diarrhea, insomnia, ringing in the ears, fatigue, bladder symptoms, anxiety, or depression.

In fact, this process of the brain generating some sensations or symptoms in the body is simply part of being human. As we shall see, our brain works to protect us from tissue damage by creating pain and it also works to "protect" us from stress and any emotional "injuries" by creating pain or other symptoms as a warning or alarm. Everyone has these reactions even if they are not aware that it is actually the brain that is causing a headache on a stressful day, a stomach ache before giving a public presentation, or a back pain when coming up to an important deadline at work.

And most importantly, this is not your fault. You are not making this up. It is not "all in your head." You are not crazy or weak. You do not want these symptoms. The symptoms you have are real, very real! They are not fake or imaginary. And, the most common cause of chronic pain is neural circuits in the brain. This means that you can get better!

The term I have used for this condition is Mind Body Syndrome, or MBS, and most people have some form of it. There are several other terms that are used to describe pain that occurs in the absence of a physical injury, such as neuroplastic or nociceptive pain syndromes and central sensitization, which are often used in scientific journals. Other commonly used terms are psychophysiologic disorders (PPD), mind-body disorders, or neural circuit disorders.

What This Program Offers

In the chapters that follow, you will learn about MBS. You will see how it can develop and why modern medicine is typically unable to solve this problem. Most importantly, you'll learn whether you suffer from this syndrome. And finally you'll be guided through a comprehensive program to cure yourself.

As a benefit of this program, you will attain increased self-awareness and greater understanding of how your brain works and of what issues in your life may have contributed to your physical pain. Not only do I expect you to be able to cure your pain, but you will be a stronger, more confident, less anxious, and less vulnerable person.

Your pain is real. But you no longer have to put up with it. This book will show you how to heal yourself. The neural circuits causing the pain can be retrained by understanding what triggers them and what amplifies them. In order to do this, we must look more closely at the brain and how it is affected by pain and by stress, and how it develops chronic pain circuits. In this way you will finally understand the underlying cause of your pain and begin to take the steps to unlearn your pain.

chapter 2

Medicine's Blind Spot

Too much light often blinds gentlemen of this sort. They cannot see the forest for the trees. — Musarion

I have about come to the conclusion that there is absolutely nothing the matter with me anyway. —Harry S. Truman, on his decision to stop pain medications for neck pain

The key to treating chronic pain and other symptoms is to determine what is causing them. This is not only good medical practice, it is common sense. However, many doctors, whether traditional or holistic, are unaware that learned neural circuits can produce a large variety of real, physical symptoms. As a result, we have a growing epidemic of pain. Many millions of people suffer, and many billions of dollars are spent on treatments that are often ineffective, such as pain medications, injections, and surgery. Despite the growing amount of money spent on treatment of these painful conditions, the results are disappointing. In fact, a study published in the *Journal of the American Medical Association* found that back and neck pain is increasing in the United States and the cost of caring for such pain has increased to more than $80 billion a year—yet the newest treatments are not any more effective than older treatments, and therefore disability due to back pain is increasing (Martin, et al., 2008). In 2011, the Institute of Medicine released a consensus report stating that approximately 110 million Americans suffer with chronic pain (Institute of Medicine, 2011). The five most common health problems causing disabilities in the US are back pain, neck pain and other musculo-skeletal pains, along with anxiety and depression (Murray, 2013).

Over the past five decades, medical science has progressed dramatically in several areas. We have made great strides in understanding and treating cancer, heart disease, stroke, hypertension, diabetes, infectious diseases, and many other illnesses. These achievements have been made to find out what is occurring on a cellular and molecular level. This approach searches for a cure by examining the specific area where the disease is found. We can see the **pathological** changes in the body in people with cancer (a tumor), heart disease (damaged heart tissue), and infections (bacteria causing tissue inflammation). But these types of physically identifiable changes cannot be found in people with Mind Body Syndrome. People with MBS do not have **pathological** changes in their body tissue; they have **physiological** changes that are reversible. That is, they have changes in blood flow, muscle tension, nerve-firing patterns, and brain-wiring patterns that create pain in the **absence** of tissue pathology.

The vast majority of physicians, including me, were trained in the biotechnological approach to medical care. We were taught: "If the back hurts, there must be something wrong with the back." We were not trained to look at the whole person to scrutinize the interaction between a person's social situation and the body, nor to examine how a patients's thoughts and emotions can affect the body.

The advances in understanding pathological processes have led us to believe that we could apply these same biotechnological approaches to chronic painful conditions that have eluded our understanding. This reductionist approach—looking at the problem solely on a tissue or molecular level—does not work when the disorder is Mind Body Syndrome. MBS is caused by a complex set of neurological connections between the brain and the body, rather than a disease localized in one area of the body.

Whiplash

Let's start with a disorder that everyone "knows" is a physical condition: whiplash. Whiplash occurs when someone is in a car accident and the head is thrown backwards, causing strain to the tendons and ligaments of the neck. The neck pain or headaches that result can last for months, years, or even decades. But does this really make sense? If you fracture a bone, you will experience significant pain for a while. But when the fracture begins to heal, the pain will subside. A whiplash injury is a sprain or a strain of the neck, certainly a less serious injury than a fracture. We wouldn't expect an ankle sprain to cause pain for years. So why wouldn't a whiplash injury heal fairly rapidly? The answer lies in the neural connections. Once these connections are fired due to the injury, they can quickly become learned. They can continue to fire and then become wired so that pain can continue for a long time, even though the ligament strain will typically heal within a week or two.

H. Schrader, a Norwegian neurologist, wondered why there were so many people on disability for whiplash in his country, so he compared the rates of whiplash in Norway to those in Lithuania. In Norway, as in the United States, if you're in a car accident, most doctors recommend rest, heat, and anti-inflammatory medications, hoping to mitigate the effects of the injury. In Lithuania, most doctors advise such patients to simply go back to work. Schrader studied 202 Lithuanians who had been in car accidents and found there were no more people with chronic headaches or neck pain than in a group that had not had car accidents. This was true even for those who had not been wearing seat belts, who had no head rests in their cars, and whose cars were severely damaged (Schrader, et. al., 1996). After this first study was criticized for gathering information after the car accidents occurred (making it a retrospective study), Dr. Schrader returned to Lithuania to conduct a prospective study, which has greater scientific validity, and he still found that whiplash did not occur there (Schrader, et. al., 2006). What we have learned is that the degree of the injury sustained is not correlated with the likelihood of developing chronic pain. Acute neck pain occurs in most injuries, but chronic pain is actually more likely to develop in those with milder rather than severe injuries (Malik and Lovell, 2004; Uomoto and Esselman, 1993).

A study by W.H. Castro and colleagues (2001) helps to give us a more complete understanding of whiplash. The researchers put fifty people in a simulation that created the sensation of having the kind of car accident that might cause whiplash. The participants had the experience of an accident, yet their necks did not move at all. Even so, 10 percent of the subjects reported neck pain four weeks after the simulated accident. Why? The researchers found that the people who developed persistent neck pain were the ones who had the most stress and emotional distress in their lives at the time of the experiment. As we shall see, their subconscious minds used the occasion of the experimental "accident" to initiate and perpetuate pain.

Without the mind at work, very few accidents and injuries would cause chronic, lasting pain. A study of demolition derby drivers revealed that almost none had chronic neck pain, even after more than 150 collisions (Simotas and Shen, 2005). Why? Because demolition derby drivers love what they do, and therefore they don't think of the collisions as traumatic. Among most people in Norway and the United States and Canada and many other countries, however, there is an expectation that if you are in a car accident, you may develop whiplash and chronic pain. And, if the accident occurs at a time in your life when there are significant stressors, the chance that chronic pain will develop is greatly increased.

JULIE, A FIFTY-FIVE-YEAR-OLD WOMAN, *had a significant car accident and was shaken up, but the doctors found no broken bones when she was seen in the emergency room. About two days later she developed neck pain, although the rest of her bruises healed and caused her no pain. Her neck, however, got worse and worse. She had X-rays and an MRI that were normal, and therefore she was told it was probably whiplash and that it could last for a long time. She had physical therapy, took painkillers, and rested—all to no avail. Her pain worsened, and she had to wear a neck collar. She stopped going out and became depressed, and the pain got so bad that she cried several times a day. About a year later, she came across Dr. John Sarno's book,* The Mindbody Prescription, *read it, and began to understand that her pain was not caused by the injuries sustained in the accident, but by a set of neural circuits that were triggered by the accident. She realized that she could get better and started doing the exercises recommended in that book. In ten days she was well enough to get rid of her neck collar, and within three weeks she was pain free. She has not had any recurrence of neck pain.*

Back Pain

The situation is very similar for the vast majority of those with back pain and sciatica. There are millions of people with chronic back pain that causes untold suffering, great expense, and huge numbers of medical procedures. Most people think that back and neck pain are degenerative disorders that will inevitably increase with increasing age. However, data from the Center for Disease Control's annual National Health Interview Survey demonstrate that back and neck pain peaks between the ages of forty-five and sixty-four and then actually declines slightly starting at age sixty-five (Strine, 2007).

Doesn't back pain mean that there is a problem in the back? Can't we see the abnormalities of the back on X-rays, CT scans, and MRIs? Actually, no, and yes. As we shall see most people with chronic back pain do not have a clearly identifiable structural abnormality to explain it. But yes, almost all people will have some sort of abnormality seen on X-rays, CT or MRI scans. To understand this, we need to look deeper at the meaning and importance of these "abnormalities."

In three separate studies by M.C. Jensen, D.G. Borenstein, and N. Boos, there was very little correlation between back pain and MRI results (Jensen, et. al., 1994; Borenstein, et. al., 2001; Boos, et. al., 2000). When you take middle-aged people **without any back pain** and give them MRIs, 60-90 percent of them have bulging discs, degenerative discs, arthritic changes, spinal stenosis, and other common changes. These findings are best interpreted as being due to normal aging, not to a disease process. If you took 100 people with back pain and 100 people without back pain and do MRIs on all of them, doctors could not look at the MRIs and predict which patients had pain and which did not. A study of healthy 21 year olds in Finland found that half of them had signs of degenerative discs and a quarter had bulging discs; all in people with no pain (Takatalo, et. al., 2009). When you take a large number of people who have no back pain at all, you find the following on

MRI Spine Imaging Findings In People With No Back Pain

	Age, n=3300						
IMAGING FINDING	**20**	**30**	**40**	**50**	**60**	**70**	**80**
DISK DEGENERATION	37%	52%	68%	80%	88%	93%	96%
DISK BULGE	30%	40%	50%	60%	69%	77%	84%
DISK PROTRUSION	29%	31%	33%	36%	38%	40%	43%
ANNULAR FISSURE	19%	20%	22%	23%	25%	27%	29%
FACET DEGENERATION	4%	9%	18%	32%	50%	69%	83%
SPONDYLOLISTHESIS	3%	5%	8%	14%	23%	35%	50%

THIS CHART SHOWS HOW COMMON THESE MRI FINDINGS ARE in people without any back pain. Even young people have relatively high rates of disk degeneration and bulging. Rates of these normal findings rise with age, yet back pain does not rise with age in the same way. The conclusion one should draw is that these findings are not actually abnormalities. They are normal signs of aging that are not the cause of pain.

Printed with permission from the American Journal of Neuroradiology
Brinjiki W, et. al. Am J Neuroradiol. 2015, 36:811-6

MRIs: 50% of healthy 30-year-olds have degenerative disc disease and 40% have bulging discs; 80% of healthy 50-year-olds have degenerative disc disease and 60% have bulging discs; and the numbers go up from there (Brinjikji, 2015).

Over time, in some people the MRI results get worse, but the pain decreases; while in others the pain gets worse, though the MRI gets better. Many people with normal MRI findings have severe back pain. In fact, Eugene Carragee of Stanford University wrote in the *New England Journal of Medicine* (2005) that "neither baseline MRIs nor follow-up MRIs are useful predictors of low back pain" and added that "ill-considered attempts to make a diagnosis on the basis of imaging studies may reinforce the suspicion of serious disease, magnify the importance of nonspecific findings, and label patients with spurious diagnoses."

If you have back pain and get an MRI, it is likely your doctor will tell you that the source of your back pain is one of the nonspecific findings Carragee warns about. Studies have shown that only 10 to 15 percent of people with back pain can be accurately diagnosed by available medical tests (Deyo, et. al., 1992). A more recent study followed over 1,100 people with acute back pain in Australia and found that only 1% of them turned out to have a significant back problem (Hensche, et. al,. 2009). Unfortunately, most physicians (whether they are neurologists, surgeons, or physical medicine specialists) and chiropractors don't heed these studies. When doctors tell a person there is a physical problem in their back based on an MRI result, the patient immediately stops being someone with back pain and starts being someone with a bad back. And if you believe you have a bad back, your pain is more likely to last longer and become more severe.

It is critically important to identify the small proportion of back pain sufferers with serious problems by the use of imaging studies. These people typically have a fracture, a tumor, or an infection and need traditional medical treatment or surgery. It is also important to have a physician examine you to make sure there is no evidence of nerve compression or damage, which is demonstrated by a change in reflexes, muscle strength, or loss of sensation. Pain that goes into an arm or leg, tingling, and numb sensations can occur due to MBS, but as long as the examination is normal, this is not clear evidence of nerve damage. At times, it is difficult to know definitively if the pain is due to MBS, or nerve damage, or a bit of both. In these situations, it is particularly helpful to have a consultation with a physician, who can conduct a thorough examination, review the records and imaging studies, and offer a reasoned opinion. Unfortunately, there are relatively few doctors who are aware of MBS. However, if your physical examination is normal and the MRI shows nothing more than the usual degenerative changes as mentioned above, then it's likely that you have MBS.

Back surgery may be necessary for some people with clear evidence of nerve damage. But without that evidence, surgery is no better than nonoperative methods for people with sciatic-type and so-called degenerative back pain, according to recent studies in the *Journal of the American Medical Association* and in the *New England Journal of Medicine* (Weinstein, et. al., 2006; Weinstein, et. al., 2007). A recent review of back pain treatment found that neither surgery, injections, or narcotic pain medications have been shown to be more effective than placebo treatments or conservative treatments (Deyo, et. al., 2009, Deyo, 2015). In particular, injections for back and neck pain are being used more often and recent studies have not found them to be more effective than placebo injections in most instances (Friedly, et. al., 2014; Staal, et. al., 2009; Chou, et. al., 2009). Even more alarming is the finding that back pain outcomes were actually worse in communities with higher rates of surgery (Keller, et. al.,1999). A study in Ohio found that 36 percent of people with job-related injuries who had back surgery had high rates of complications, and 27 percent had repeat operations. The return-to-work rate was 66 percent in those who did not have surgery compared to 26 percent for those who had back surgery (Nguyen, et. al., 2011). If you or someone you know is considering surgery for back pain, I strongly recommend reading *Back in Control* by my colleague and spine surgeon, Dr. David Hanscom and *Watch Your Back* by Dr. Richard Deyo. Finally, there is emerging evidence that treatment of chronic pain with narcotic analgesics can actually worsen pain, because narcotics can increase nerve sensitization (Mitra, 2008; Silverman, 2009).

I routinely see people with severe and chronic back pain (including many who were taking morphine or Vicodin or who were on the verge of back surgery) who have had dramatic results in a very short time by using this treatment program for Mind Body Syndrome.

HELEN, A SIXTY-FIVE-YEAR-OLD WOMAN, *had suffered from nine years of back pain. The pain started in her lower back one day while she was working at her job on an automobile assembly line. It was so severe that she had to be carried out of the factory. She was seen by several doctors, and eventually an MRI revealed the following:*

Severe disc space narrowing at L4-L5 and flattened discs at L2-L3 and L3-L4. Disc bulging with flattening of the spinal cord and narrowing of the outlet for the spinal nerves at L2-L3, L3-L4, L4-L5, and L5-S1. The right L4 and L5 nerve roots are compressed by a disc. The facet joints are swollen and there is spinal stenosis.

Helen underwent seven courses of physical therapy, along with massage therapy, acupuncture, electrode nerve stimulation, and specialty care from a pain management clinic. Despite these treatments, her pain continued. It radiated to her right leg and heel, and she began to develop numbness in her left thigh. After nine years on disability leave she finally took an early retirement, and a neurosurgeon scheduled her for lumbar fusion surgery due to the chronic and severe pain. Her physical exam showed normal reflexes, normal muscle strength, and normal sensation despite her symptoms of pain and numbness.

Helen was the oldest of ten siblings. Her father beat her when she was a child, and her mother required her to do a great deal of housework and child care. She recalls going into a closet and screaming, "I hate my parents! I hate my parents!" She had a difficult adult life, which included raising three children by herself, three divorces, and struggles with alcoholism (though Alcoholics Anonymous had helped her remain sober for twenty-seven years). She had many financial difficulties and became very unhappy with her job.

By participating in this program, Helen noted marked pain relief over the first two weeks. The numbness in her thigh disappeared. By the end of the four-week program, she was pain free and canceled her back surgery. Her joy was incalculable, and she felt in control of her body and her life for the first time in nine years.

Four months later, she had a recurrence of back pain one day, but she quickly figured out what caused it. It began on the day she learned that her daughter was scheduled to depart for military duty in Iraq. Recognizing that her emotional stress was responsible for this pain, she used the methods taught in the program to rapidly rid herself of the pain. "In the past, stress would cause pain in my body that would cripple me," Helen said. "But now I look at it, and it goes away."

KATHERINE, A FORTY-TWO-YEAR-OLD WOMAN, *came to me with four years of left buttock and leg pain. Her pain began in the area of her left hamstring while she was running in a ten-kilometer "fun run," an easy task for an active person who had previously run marathons and had regularly hiked, skied, and mountain biked. Despite rest and anti-inflammatory agents, the pain worsened. She then received physical therapy, chiropractic treatments, acupuncture, and massage; she also tried yoga, pilates, and Rolfing, with no improvement.*

MRI scans of her back and X-rays of her hip were normal, and Katherine was diagnosed by different physicians as having a pulled hamstring, iliotibial band syndrome, sacroiliac joint instability, and a leg length discrepancy. Despite all of the above therapies, the pain persisted and spread to her hip, outer thigh, and gluteal area. She stopped running and could not do any other physical activities because of the pain. After being seen by a family physician, orthopedic physician, neurologist, and physical medicine specialist with no improvement, Katherine was eventually referred to a nationally renowned medical center. There, she was given a diagnosis of piriformis syndrome and received a steroid injection followed by more physical therapy. Unfortunately, her pain did not diminish, and Katherine continued to spend significant portions of each day in bed or lying on the couch. Over the last few years, she had developed pain in her right scapular area and her right hip as well.

Katherine had experienced tension and migraine headaches as an adolescent. She also suffered from insomnia, fatigue, and depression when she was in her early thirties after her father and mother divorced. Katherine noted multiple stressors over the past several years: she had moved to a new city, her husband had started a new job, her mother had suffered a heart attack, her child had trouble sleeping, and she had renovated her husband's office and her home. She admitted to having high expectations of herself, frequently feeling guilty and being overly conscientious. She told me that she had all but given up on all of her dreams and abilities to live a normal life because of her great pain.

By participating in this program, Katherine was able to connect the occurrence of pain with her life experiences. Her pain diminished within the first two weeks of the program, and she began to resume her normal activities, including running twice a week without pain. After four weeks, she wrote, "I am so happy to say that I now have the ability to recognize that my pain is caused by an accumulation of anger and guilt in my mind and that it uses my body as its outlet and that I no longer allow it to do so. This has taken work on my part; however, I am thankful that I am able to now let go and be pain free."

Fibromyalgia

One of the more enigmatic disorders is fibromyalgia, which means "painful muscles and tissues." People diagnosed with this disorder have chronic widespread pain throughout their bodies, but no one can tell them why. Despite great efforts to find a structural cause, there is no pathological process (no tissue breakdown or destruction) in the bones, joints, tendons, or muscles, yet the pain can be severe and debilitating. Brain imaging studies have shown that the pain is real and is felt as much as pain from a bone fracture (Gracely, et. al., 2002). It is incredibly frustrating for people with widespread pain to have no idea what causes it, to be considered crazy by some, to be considered incurable by others, and to get little or no relief from available pain medications, muscle relaxants, anti-depressants, and mood stabilizers (Wolfe, 2009; Baumgartner, et. al., 2002; Goldenberg, 2004). Because of the difficulties in understanding and treating fibromyalgia, people who suffer with this very real and often severely painful condition have often been treated poorly by the medical profession. Having been told many times that their pain is "all in their head," patients are understandably sensitive to any psychological interventions. Few patients and even fewer doctors realize that real pain can be caused by stress and unresolved emotions. If you are skeptical of this concept, you're not alone. However, keep an open mind as you read the next few chapters and I believe you will begin to be convinced. If you are, you have the opportunity to free yourself from this horrible disorder.

People with fibromyalgia also commonly have lower back pain, migraine or tension headaches, temporomandibular joint (TMJ) pain, irritable bowel and bladder syndromes, insomnia, brain fog or many of the other Mind Body Syndrome symptoms (Geisser, et. al., 2008). Biomedical experts have been able to determine that there is sensitization of neural circuits in the brains of people with fibromyalgia and changes in some of the neurotransmitters in their brains (Yunus, 2007). However, they have not been able to develop any significant breakthrough medical therapies. In fact, very few patients with this condition have been cured or gone into remission through standard medical treatments (Walitt, et. al., 2011).

There is ample evidence that people with fibromyalgia have much higher rates of life stressors and victimization (physical, sexual, or emotional abuse) compared to people with other physical disorders and compared to the general population (Goldberg, et. al., 1999; van Houdenhove, et. al., 2001). There is also a large overlap between those with fibromyalgia and those experiencing anxiety, depression, and post-traumatic stress disorder (Cohen, et. al., 2002; Celiker, et. al., 1997). As we shall see in the next chapter, the effects of these stressors are the cause of the painful fibromyalgia symptoms. However, most physicians and researchers can only offer medications to try to cover up the pain. These medications do not lead to cures because they don't get to the root of the problem.

I have seen many people released from the pain of this disorder using the program outlined in this book. If you listen carefully to the full life history of people with fibromyalgia, it becomes crystal clear that it's a form of MBS. In fact, I have conducted research to determine how effective this program is for fibromyalgia, and the results have been gratifying (Hsu, et. al., 2010). Six weeks after their MBS treatment, approximately 25 percent of patients have gone into remission, meaning their pain has been eliminated or reduced to very low levels. Another 25 percent have experienced a moderate reduction in their pain. These results may not seem remarkable, but consider this: These reductions in pain are long lasting (measured at six months) and exceed the results found in studies of medications. The women with fibromyalgia who were in the control group in this research study were able to use any medications or other treatments. However, none of them showed any evidence of pain reduction. In a more recent study, conducted with my colleague, Mark Lumley, PhD, we demonstrated even better results. We studied a group of 75 individuals who had a history of chronic pain for an average of 8.8 years and whose primary disorder was fibromyalgia or back pain, although most patients had many symptoms of MBS. Their average baseline pain scores were 5.1 on a 10-point scale and 57% had a history of significant childhood trauma. Six months after going through the Mind Body program, 53% showed a reduction in average pain scores by at least 50% and 67% had at least a 30% reduction in pain scores. These are remarkable results for people who have suffered with pain for so many years (Burger A, et. al., 2016). This program requires you to fully understand this model, believe that it applies to you, and be fully committed to the process. People with fibromyalgia and other chronic painful conditions who do these things almost always obtain significant results in this program.

In a larger study funded by the National Institutes of Health, Mark Lumley and I compared the kinds of treatments used in this book to the standard psychological treatment for fibromyalgia pain, cognitive-behavioral therapy (CBT) in a randomized, controlled trial. We found that this treatment, emotional awareness and expression therapy (EAET, which is described later in this book) was more effective than CBT in reducing pain. Approximately 22% of those treated with EAET had more than 50% pain reduction at a six-month follow up compared to about 9% of those treated with CBT. This was one of the first studies to show that one psychological treatment for pain was actually better than another (Lumley, 2017). In a more recent study, Brandon Yarns showed that veterans with chronic musculo-skeletal pain had more benefits from EAET than from CBT, with 31% of those having greater than 50% pain reduction compared to none in the CBT group (Yarns, et. al., 2020).

ANJANI, A FORTY-SEVEN-YEAR-OLD WOMAN *who migrated to the United States from India, reached a point in her life when she was beginning to think of doing some more things for herself, such as taking classes at a local college. However, her husband took an extra job, and she had three adolescent children who required a lot of her time. On top of that, her mother-in-law moved into her house and began to lecture her on how to be a better cook, homemaker, and mother. In addition, her brother moved in and expected her to wait on him. Being a dutiful person who put her obligations to others ahead of her own desires, she complied with these additional stressful tasks and cancelled her class, but she had no outlet for her feelings of resentment. Her body reacted to these stresses and suppressed emotions with a widespread painful process, which was labeled as fibromyalgia. After going through this program, her pain was dramatically reduced. One of the keys to her improvement was that she decided to speak up for herself and take more control over her situation at home.*

JANET, A FORTY-ONE-YEAR-OLD WOMAN, *grew up with a mother who was emotionally distant. The mother was very busy with her own life and was usually gone, often playing bridge and tennis. Janet had no illnesses or symptoms of MBS until she was in her thirties. She was happily married, with two small children, for whom she was determined to be the best mother possible. She was having a new home built and trying to make it perfect. At this time, she began to develop widespread pain in her muscles and tendons, which was diagnosed as fibromyalgia. When I asked her what her mother was doing at the time she and her children needed her help, she replied, "Playing bridge and tennis." She then began to sob over the loss that she experienced as a child and that her children were now experiencing. Her mother was being as distant with her grandchildren as she had been with her own daughter. At this stressful point in her life, that separation was enough to trigger severe pain in her body. Once she realized that she was not physically ill and that her pain came from unexpressed emotions, her pain totally disappeared.*

Headaches and Other Disorders

Tension headaches and migraine headaches afflict millions of people in the United States. More and more people are suffering, and specialized headache clinics have been established for people with severe symptoms. Yet, despite the development of many new medications, we see rising costs of treatment as well as increased loss of productivity due to absences from work and school.

The vast majority of people with chronic headaches have normal CT scans and MRIs. Tests do not detect anything wrong in their brains. As with fibromyalgia, there are many theories about what causes these headaches, from food and chemical sensitivities to genetics. Such things can trigger headaches, but they are not the main underlying cause of these severe and chronic headaches. Let me briefly explain, but there will be much more on this topic later in the book. We have learned that many people have triggers to pain that can be unlearned. For example, if changes in the weather or certain foods or certain movements or activities trigger migraine or other pains, it is likely that these factors are simply causing the brain to activate the neural circuits for pain, rather than actually causing a physical reaction due to an injury. This is known as a conditioned response, which is reversible. Migraine is a good example of a disorder that can have a genetic predisposition. In other words, people with family members who have it may have genes that make it more likely to occur. This is also the case with genes for depression. However, it is important to understand that these genes function in an epigenetic manner, meaning that the genes can actually be turned on and off by life stresses. Therefore people with migraine can get better despite having a genetic predisposition for it by using this program.

Headache specialists do not generally listen very carefully to a patient's life story. Even if they did, they may not be aware that mental events can produce such severe symptoms. When you look very carefully at the onset of headaches and at the precise times they worsen, you will find that conscious and/or subconscious emotions are at the root of the problem.

VICKIE, A FIFTY-FIVE-YEAR-OLD WOMAN, *suffered from constant daily headaches for seventeen years. She had been evaluated by twenty doctors and had been placed on more than twenty different medications in an attempt to control the persistent pain. She had even had a surgical procedure to attempt to relieve pressure on a facial nerve that was thought to be trapped by muscles.*

She had never had headaches until the day when she put on a new pair of prescription glasses and instantly developed pain on the left side of her head that radiated into her face. The pain worsened over the years, and no treatment ever helped.

When I listened carefully to her life story, she told me that her mother was aloof and her father was "bipolar" and unpredictable. Some days, he would come home from work and be fine, but on many occasions he would be in a bad mood and would often grab her by her collar and scream at her. Despite this difficult upbringing, she had no symptoms at all as a child.

At the time when Vickie got the glasses, her home life was fine. However, she had recently gotten a new boss, a woman whom she described as "mean and nasty," who would frequently scream at her.

It became obvious that the new glasses did not cause her headaches, but when she put them on, her subconscious mind used the opportunity to create pain in the same way that a real or simulated car accident can become an opportunity for pain of whiplash. Vickie quit her job a few months later, but by that time the vicious cycle of nerve connections had been formed, and her headaches continued on a daily basis. She started this program, and her headaches gradually began to decrease. After the program, her headaches continued to improve, and after six months she became free of them altogether.

There are several other conditions that are typically manifestations of MBS, such as chronic abdominal pain and pelvic pain, TMJ pain, irritable bowel syndrome, irritable bladder syndrome (known as interstitial cystitis), chronic fatigue, tinnitus, insomnia, anxiety and depression. See the

Conditions that are Commonly Caused By Mind Body Syndrome

CHRONIC PAIN SYNDROMES

Tension headaches

Migraine headaches

Back pain

Neck pain

Whiplash

Fibromyalgia

Temporomandibular joint (TMJ) syndrome

Chronic abdominal and pelvic pain syndromes

Chronic tendonitis

Vulvodynia

Piriformis syndrome

Sciatic pain syndrome

Repetitive stress injury

Foot pain syndromes

Myofascial pain syndrome

AUTONOMIC NERVOUS SYSTEM RELATED DISORDERS

Irritable bowel syndrome

Interstitial cystitis (Irritable bladder syndrome)

Postural orthostatic tachycardia syndrome

Inappropriate sinus tachycardia

Reflex sympathetic dystrophy (Complex regional pain syndrome, CRPS)

Functional dyspepsia

OTHER SYNDROMES

Insomnia

Chronic fatigue syndrome

Paresthesias (numbness, tingling, burning)

Tinnitus

Dizziness

Spasmodic dysphonia

Chronic hives

Anxiety

Depression

Obsessive-compulsive disorder

Post-traumatic stress disorder

Multiple chemical sensitivities

NOTE: *Many of the symptoms in this table can be caused by physical disorders that require medical treatment. Consult your doctor or a specialist in Mind Body Medicine (see the Appendix) to determine if you can participate in this program. See Chapter 5 for help in determining if you have Mind Body Syndrome.*

table on page 20 for a list of common syndromes caused by MBS. This list of symptoms includes those that are commonly encountered by doctors like myself who see patients with Mind Body Syndrome. However, almost any symptom can be caused by MBS, just as any symptom can be caused by a medical or structural problem. Over the years, I have seen people with a variety of unusual symptoms that are due to MBS, such as burning of the mouth, ears, hands, or feet, tingling or electric sensations of almost any body part. Sensations caused by the brain are real, they are caused by neural circuits that are real; they can be powerful and we experience them in a very real way. However, if we can understand that MBS sensations are not dangerous, that our brain is producing them, we can then be much more confident in taking the necessary steps to reduce or eliminate them. We can change these neural circuits and that is the basis of this book. If a careful medical evaluation does not show any clear pathologic process, then the symptoms in these conditions are likely caused by a vicious cycle of nerve connections that have been learned by the mind and body.

Standard Treatment Equals Faulty Diagnosis

What happens if you develop any of these MBS symptoms and seek care from your physician? The doctor will rarely take a careful enough history to determine if the symptoms may be related to stressful events and emotions. However, your doctor will usually do thorough medical testing to look for serious disorders such as cancer, immune disorders, fractures, and heart and vascular diseases. These tests are very important to make sure you don't have a tissue breakdown disease. If the tests find no clear evidence of disease, you may become more anxious because there is no clear explanation for the symptoms, and the doctor may be puzzled and tell you that the pain is all in your head. This is one of the worst things a doctor can say to someone. Mind Body Syndrome is a real condition, and it can be effectively treated. It is not imaginary or brought on because the patient wants to be sick. Many people that I see are frustrated with their doctors for not explaining what is going on and why they are in pain. The reason most doctors don't adequately explain chronic pain is that they don't understand this disorder.

If the doctor finds something on an MRI such as a degenerating disc or bulging disc or spinal stenosis, the patient will often be led to believe there is a serious medical condition. Once someone is told that they have fibromyalgia, they may be initially relieved to discover that there is a name for their severe symptoms. However, once they are told that they will have to manage the pain since there are no effective treatments to cure it, they are likely to become upset and depressed.

Traditional medical treatments are geared towards correcting the underlying pathology in the body. In MBS, there are reversible physiological changes to the brain and nerve pathways, but there is no underlying tissue breakdown. Standard treatments don't address the true cause of these symptoms but try to cover them up. Pain medications, migraine medications, stomach and bladder medications, physical therapy, acupuncture, vitamins, herbs, and all of the other therapies recommended for these disorders will often provide at most a partial or a temporary relief. When these therapies and medications do work for people with MBS, it is usually due to the placebo effect, that is, the expectation by the patient that the treatment will work (Bausell, 2007; Brody and Brody, 2001). With this belief, the mind allows the treatment to work—but often the relief is only temporary, since the person has not understood what caused the problem in the first place.

Despite the absence of confirmed pathology, the doctor will often make a diagnosis. Medicine has given names to these clusters of symptoms: fibromyalgia, migraine headaches, sciatica, interstitial cystitis, TMJ disorder. This labeling is often harmful. The patient now thinks he or she has a serious condition, and websites for these conditions support the belief that the condition could be severe and long lasting. If referred to a pain clinic, patients are often told that they have a disorder called "chronic pain" and that the goal of their treatment will be to help them be more functional, rather than to reduce their pain. Even the top pain clinics and pain rehabilitation programs in the country take this position: that chronic pain is incurable and that the best we can do is to help people cope with it better. When no clear physical cause is found, the diagnosis given will often be central sensitization, meaning that the brain has sensitized pain circuits that are persistently firing, and that it is irreversible. Psychological treatments such as CBT, acceptance and commitment therapy, and mindfulness based therapies, are all excellent approaches, but they have limited value when they are used for coping, rather than curing. From my point of view, pain is a symptom of an underlying process. It is not a diagnosis any more than a fever is. With pain and fever and other symptoms, there are underlying causes.

The medical profession has unwittingly created a form of mental imprisonment called medicalization, when diagnosis and treatment causes an increase in pain and suffering. The false belief that one has a serious and intractable condition causes activation of more stress and emotional reactions, such as depression, hopelessness, helplessness, fear, and anxiety, that can exacerbate the problem. This is known as the nocebo effect, where the subconscious brain begins to "expect" that things will get worse, and then the brain activates increases in neural circuit based symptoms. When MBS is treated as a purely physical condition, the symptoms often get worse rather than getting better. Injections, pain medications, and surgery can cause side effects and even be dangerous at times. In addition, the cost associated with such faulty diagnoses are staggering. It is estimated that up to one third of the medical care in the U.S. is unnecessary (Brownlee, 2007).

The first critical step in dealing with chronic symptoms is to get the correct diagnosis. If there is a tissue breakdown disorder, then I would recommend traditional medical treatments. If you have been suffering for some time, if your doctors haven't been able to adequately explain why you have so much pain, if your only options are surgery or pain medications, then you are likely to have MBS. If the true diagnosis is Mind Body Syndrome, then traditional medical therapies are not likely to cure the condition. Your doctors have not been able to help you because they have been looking in the wrong place.

chapter 3

How Pain Develops: The Role of the Brain

Human beings owe a surprisingly large proportion of their cognitive and behavioral capacities to the existence of an "automatic self" of which they have no conscious knowledge and over which they have little voluntary control. — Jonathan Miller

Why do so many people have pain and other symptoms caused by Mind Body Syndrome? How do the brain and the body learn the vicious cycle of pain? The key to understanding the answers is to recognize how the brain works and how stress and emotions play a vital role in the initiation and perpetuation of pain.

We live in a stressful world to which we have not fully adapted. Our brains are wired to react to the very different, ancient world of our ancestors. They experienced acute stress—for example, dangerous animals—on an occasional basis. In those situations, the brain activates the powerful fight-or-flight reaction to deal with the acute stress, the body becomes tense, and after that stress is over (assuming the individual survives unharmed), the body relaxes. The brain is well programmed to deal with that kind of acute stress. However, the brain often has trouble dealing with the chronic stress of modern life. That's why, when stress becomes chronic and we feel trapped in situations for which there is no easy way out, we can easily develop a set of neural circuits that are painful.

You already know that stress causes physical reactions. Your face will turn red if you are embarrassed. That's because your emotions cause the autonomic nervous system to increase blood flow to the face. This is a very real bodily response to an emotion. If you have a stressful day at work or at school, you might get a headache; this is also real pain caused by emotions. If you have to give a speech in front of hundreds of people, your stomach may tighten up from nervousness. These are normal everyday reactions caused by the connections between the brain and the body. Everyone accepts that these are physical reactions to stressful events, that they are not signs of disease, and that the symptoms will disappear when the stress that triggers them subsides.

This is exactly the mechanism of Mind Body Syndrome: Stress triggers emotions that cause our bodies to react by producing physical symptoms. The symptoms are real. Your face really does turn red when you blush from embarrassment. Your head or your stomach really does hurt if you've had a difficult day or face a daunting challenge. The symptoms, including the pain, are not imaginary. They are physical processes. They are real. But they are physiological processes that can be reversed. They are temporary.

If you have these symptoms, you're not crazy. You're normal. Almost everyone has some physical symptoms due to the body's reaction to stress. I have asked hundreds of people during my lectures if they know where they "hold" stress in their bodies, and almost everyone has an answer. It is common knowledge that stress can cause physical reactions.

What is not common knowledge is that stress and emotions can create the neural circuits that can cause chronic and often severe physical symptoms. What is also not commonly known is that it is the brain that actually creates all pain, as we shall see. The cure for such chronic pain or other symptoms is not a drug or a remedy designed to lessen or cover up these symptoms. If you do not find and treat the underlying cause of the pain, you will not get better. For most people, the underlying cause is that neural circuits have been activated that actually create physical pain. There are several methods of training the brain out of that pain that are contained in this book.

The Emotional Brain

The way our brains work explains how the stresses of life can turn into bodily pain. Though our brains are very complicated and everyone reacts differently to stresses, we share many things in common. We all need to be loved, nurtured, and protected. We all need to grow, develop, and become independent. We all have thoughts and emotions and memories.

Our emotional memories are imprinted in our brains and stored in what are called associative networks (LeDoux, 1996). They are imprinted in a network of the brain that registers and stores emotions, which includes several structures such as the amygdala, hippocampus, insula, anterior cingulate cortex and prefrontal cortex. These areas are closely connected to the hypothalamus, the center for the autonomic nervous system (ANS) (van der Kolk, 1994; Okifuji and Turk, 2002). The ANS controls our breathing, heart rate, blood pressure, temperature, and many other automatic and involuntary functions—the things our body does without our conscious mind being aware of them.

During times of stress, the emotion-based network sends signals to activate the ANS and produce the hormones cortisol and adrenaline, which turn on the "fight or flight" reaction. That's a system that directs blood flow to muscles to get our body ready to run or do battle, and it causes our bodies to react instantly before we are aware of what is going on. Human beings have this system to protect us from danger and improve our chances for survival.

If we see something squiggly moving across the ground, our brain activates the autonomic nervous system and causes us to immediately jump back to protect ourselves. We do not stop and reach out to see what the squiggly thing is. That conscious action could get us killed. Our protective system kicks in before we have the chance to think. In fact, research shows that when emotions arise quickly, the blood flow in the brain shifts away from the frontal lobes, the conscious thinking part of the brain, to the limbic system, which is the emotional, reacting, and subconscious part of the brain, which includes the amygdala and the autonomic nervous system (Takamatsu, et. al., 2003).

The Role of the Autonomic Nervous System

The autonomic nervous system controls the nerve fibers that affect every area of your body. Studies have shown that emotions such as anxiety or anger cause increased tension in the back muscles of people with chronic back pain (Burns, et. al., 2006; Quartana and Burns, 2007). This muscle tension, which typically takes place without our conscious awareness, can cause real and severe physical pain. Often we are not even aware of the emotions that are triggering these automatic physical responses, which is why they are referred to as subconscious or unconscious emotions.

There is a large variety of processes that can occur with ANS activation. Not only are muscles and blood flow involved, but the nervous system, the heart, the gastrointestinal (GI) system, and the genitourinary (GU) systems can all be altered. And the ANS can produce very specific changes, depending on the specific situation, that will vary from person to person and from moment to moment (Levenson, 1992; Burns, et. al., 2008). A careful understanding of the reactions of animals to stressful situations reveals that they may fight or flee, but they may also freeze (as a rabbit will do) or submit (play dead) (LeDoux, 1996). The ANS can produce a much greater variety of symptoms in response to stress and emotional reactions in humans. Activation of the muscles can produce pain in almost any part of the body. Nervous system activation can produce tingling, numbness, or burning sensations as well as dizziness, tinnitus, and anxiety. Activation of the GI system can cause abdominal pain or bloating, heartburn, nausea and vomiting, diarrhea or constipation. When the GU system is activated, one can experience pain, itching, burning, and urinary frequency. Cardiovascular (CV) activation can produce palpitations and a rapid heart rate. Alterations in blood flow can produce migraine headaches. And the freeze and submission responses typically cause fatigue and/or depression. It is important to realize that the ANS is not acting on its own. It is controlled by the brain and the danger/alarm mechanism that can turn on or turn off these autonomic physical responses.

Pain caused by ANS activation can occur suddenly with an acute spasm of muscles, or it can develop gradually over time. It can occur in the back, neck, head, abdomen, pelvis, or almost anywhere in the body. This pain can be constant or occasional, it can be mild or severe, and it can feel like an ache, a numbness, or a shooting pain. For people who suffer in these various ways in various places because of Mind Body Syndrome, there is no tissue breakdown or physical disease in the body. Yet, the pain is real. As we shall see, the pain is caused by an activation of a neural circuit..

Pain in the Brain

The brain has complex mechanisms to handle pain that involves many structures. The neuroscientists commonly refer to this network as a "salience network," meaning that the brain decides what is most salient (or more important) for it to attend to (Barrett and Simmons, 2015). If you are running from a lion and twist your ankle, your brain will likely not activate pain so that you have the best chance of escaping. However, if one of our ancestors was running after a deer and broke his ankle, the brain would want to create severe pain so that he would immediately stop and rest the foot in order to heal. If pain did not occur in that situation, he would continue running and could completely destroy the ankle leading to long-term disability. Our subconscious brains decide when to turn on pain and when to turn it off, by activating this salience network that we commonly call the danger/alarm mechanism.

The subconscious controls not only responses to our environment but also what we perceive. Eyewitness accounts are dramatically altered by the values and experiences of the viewer (Arkowitz and Lilienfeld, 2010; Drew, et. al., 2013; Lum, et. al., 2005). We can see only what our brains expect us to see. This is known as predictive processing: what we perceive is predicted from past experiences. For visual, auditory and taste perceptions, this is termed exteroception. Over time, we learn to like and dislike certain music and foods. A similar process, interoception, occurs for internal sensations (Barrett and Simmons, 2015): The brain creates the sensations it expects us to feel. When the brain is in an ongoing state of warning or danger, it will continue to produce pain with movement, fatigue with activity, disordered thought processes, and many other sensations designed to enforce rest and inactivity. And the more the accompanying neural circuits are activated, they more they become normalized as default circuits.

I have learned that it's very important to truly understand how the brain creates all of our internal experiences in order to understand pain and other symptoms. Let's review that in detail here.

The term neuroscientists are now using to describe how the brain works is predictive coding or predictive processing. This means that our brain doesn't just react to our environment, but that the brain actively helps us navigate the world by trying to predict what will happen next so that we are prepared for it. It's like a soccer goalie trying to figure out how the opposing player will kick a penalty kick. The goalie has to guess which way the ball will go. Sometimes, they get it right and can make the save, but sometimes they get it wrong, and the ball sails into the net.

How do we see?

Actually, we do not see with our eyes, we see with our brains. Light comes into our eyes, but the actual images that we see are made (or constructed) in a part of the brain called the visual cortex (towards the back of the brain). Most of the nerve fibers that go to our visual cortex do not come from our eyes, but come from within the brain itself. These fibers transmit information from our memories of what people, cars, trees and birds look like.

If I had you wear prism glasses that turned all images upside down, you would see everything upside down. But not for long! In a few hours or a day or two, your brain would convert those images right side up again, even though the light waves are still upside down. If you look straight ahead and close one eye and then the other eye, you will see the same image in front of you. That's because your brain is using both eyes to see at the same time. But if you keep your head straight and look all the way to your right side, you will be looking out of the "corner of your eye." Then close your left eye; you will still see the same image to your right side. But if you close your right eye, you will see an image in front of you, not to the side. This means that your brain has automatically turned off the images coming into your visual cortex from your left eye. It is only using the images from your right eye. Smart brain!

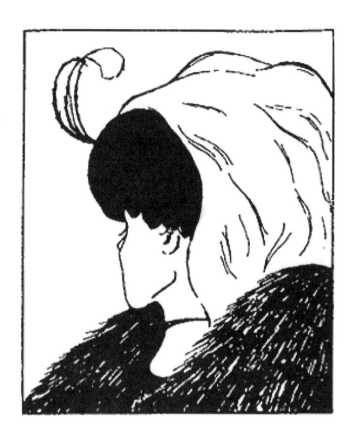

It is always working to help you navigate the world.

Look at this image. What do you see? Do you see one or two women? They are looking in different directions and one is younger and the other more "mature." Vision is constructed in the brain and your brain will be able to see both of these images once you have looked at this long enough. After a bit, it will be easy to see each of the images as your brain has made the neural connections or circuits for seeing those images. And you will probably be able to switch from one image (one neural circuit) to the other image (a different neural circuit) by choosing which image to pay attention to. This is an example of how our brains work, by activating different neural circuits and then paying more attention to one of them than to another.

Police officers have very difficult jobs at times. They are called to uncertain and potentially dangerous situations, and their brain is continually asking this question: "Do I see a gun or not?" And it's stressful, and there is very little time for actual consideration. So, what happens? Sometimes, the officer is accurate about whether the people they meet have a gun or not; and sometimes, their brain will actually see a gun that is not there, or vice versa.

How do we hear? With our ears? Well, not actually. A couple of years ago, a young woman got up to give a presentation at our hospital and she said: "Good morning, America." That seemed odd, but that's what I heard. In reality, she said "Good morning, I'm Erica." But I didn't know her name and my brain was just trying to make sense of the sounds, so it came up with something that was familiar to me from US television.

Have you ever heard someone call your name, yet find out that no one had? This is common and has happened to me.

Our brain is constantly working to predict what we will need and then to create that experience. The simple act of standing up is actually very complex: your heart rate will increase a bit, the blood vessels going to the brain will dilate to create more blood flow to the brain, many different muscle groups will be activated, the balance center will be put into gear. All of those things happen immediately and effortlessly, all occurring due to actions by the brain. And, most importantly, these actions occur before you actually stand up. Your brain anticipates (predicts) what you will need and creates that experience ahead of time so that it is there, waiting for you to actually stand up. The same kinds of actions occur every time you walk up or down a flight of steps.

If you are thirsty, your brain will start turning off the sensation of thirst before you drink that glass of water. If you have a slight headache due to missing your morning coffee, your brain will turn off the headache as soon as you pick up that warm cup of joe.

Have you ever felt your cell phone vibrating in your pocket when it wasn't? This is also common and has also happened to me.

So, it turns out that all of the sensations that we feel in our bodies are actually created by our brains. There are literally millions of inputs from every spot of our body that are going to the brain each second. Our brain has to decide which ones to ignore and which ones to pay attention to. If our lungs, heart and kidneys are working fine at the moment, no need to pay attention to them and no need for the brain to create a sensation to alert us to some kind of problem there.

A few years ago, my wife woke up early while I was still in bed and got her usual breakfast: sliced apples, yogurt and granola. That day, she had an extra slice and brought it to the bedroom, which was still dark and fed it to me. I didn't see it or touch it before biting on it. As soon as I bit on it, I got a rotten taste in my mouth, as if I was eating a rotten apple. But I wasn't. That day, my wife had a peach, instead of an apple.

My brain was expecting an apple; predicting a certain sensation arriving from the body. When it got the softness of the peach instead of the crunch of an apple, it immediately reacted to protect me, giving me a rotten taste with the message: "Don't eat that, spit it out, it's dangerous/poisonous." My brain ignored the sweet taste of the peach (and I love peaches) and replaced that sweet taste with a rotten one. That is predictive processing in action. All of our sensations are actually created by the brain, whether it's taste, touch, pain, anxiety, what we see and what we hear.

Pain is one of the brain's ways of protecting us. It is a powerful mechanism to give us a strong sign of something being wrong. If you are running across a field and you break an ankle, do you want pain? Of course you do! If you didn't get pain, you would keep running on a broken ankle, which would even more severely damage that ankle. We know that all pain is basically protective. It protects us from further harm by alerting us to the danger. In fact, children who are born without the ability to feel pain often have severe injuries and may die at a young age.

Amazingly, it is not the broken ankle that causes pain, but rather the brain's danger/alarm signal. It alerts you and forces you to stop running, so that you can rest and heal. The broken ankle will activate nerve signals that go to the brain, but it is the brain that will "decide" whether to actually turn on pain or not!

But what if you were running across a field being chased by a lion and you broke an ankle? Would you want pain then? Probably not, as you would die if you got pain, so in that case, as mentioned, the brain would probably make a decision to not turn on pain so that you could try to escape with your life. Pain is a decision made by the brain on a moment by moment basis.

To repeat, when we cut our finger or touch a hot stove, it is not the finger causing pain. It is the brain. Nerve impulses from the finger are sent to the brain immediately, but it is the brain that turns on pain. Or not. Sometimes, we can get injured and the brain does not turn on pain. There are hundreds of stories about this. In fact, a study of soldiers from World War II found that a majority of those who were injured did not describe any pain once they got into the safety of a medical unit.

A friend of mine was alone at a construction site when he accidentally shot a nail into his hand. Shockingly, he had no pain at all! No pain with a nail sticking into his hand. For some reason, his brain "decided" not to turn on pain at that moment, despite the obvious injury. Why? Well, we don't know since the brain just acts and reacts to situations as best as it can. We can guess that a millisecond decision by his brain factored in two options: 1) Be in severe pain, all alone at a construction site, or 2) Create no pain and let him drive himself to the hospital for help. It chose #2.

It's important to understand that we have absolutely no control (or very little control) over these critical, rapid decisions made by the brain. The brain works primarily on a subconscious basis, i.e., we are unaware of all of these decisions and actions. We just know that they occur, after they occur!

Now you know that not all injuries cause pain. Pain is a decision made by the brain. What about the opposite situation? Can the brain create pain when there is no injury at all? Not only can it do that, but this is an extremely common occurrence, even though few people are aware of it.

To see some amazing demonstrations of neural circuits in the brain, go to unlearnyourpain.com, click on the Media tab at the top of the home page, select videos and watch the Rubber Arm and the Backwards Bicycle videos.

How the Brain Creates Pain

The fact that pain can be felt in an area that is not diseased has been illustrated in phantom limb syndrome, where an amputee experiences pain that feels like it is coming from the part of the body that's been amputated. Phantom limb syndrome is a perfect example of Mind Body Syndrome—pain is felt in an area that is clearly not diseased. The pain is caused by nerve sensitization and brain reorganization producing pain, which is felt in the missing limb (Flor, et. al., 1995).

Going one step further, a group of researchers tried to determine if the brain could actually create pain (Derbyshire, et. al., 2004). They took a group of people and exposed them to three distinct conditions; thermal pain in one hand, the hypnotic suggestion that they were feeling thermal hand pain, and simply imagining feeling thermal hand pain while not under hypnosis. Their brains were imaged to see if there were differences between these three conditions. The brain images showed that similar areas were activated in the thermal pain and the hypnotic pain situations (including the ACC and a few other areas), while fewer and different brain areas were activated during imagined pain. This was the first evidence that the brain can create pain that is indistinguishable from pain caused by stimulation of nerves in tissues. This research helps confirm that real pain can be caused by either physical disease states or by neuroplastic processes that create learned neural circuits, as with a psychophysiologic disorder. The fact is that all pain is experienced in the brain. We cannot have pain without activation of the pain pathways in the brain. As we shall see, the brain can turn off pain even when the body is injured or has some degree of tissue damage. And, as just mentioned, pain can occur when there is no physical injury or tissue damage. This type of pain is very common. When I was explaining this to one of my patients, she smiled and said, "Oh, I get it. The pain isn't in my head; it's in my brain!" With that understanding, she took a huge step in the process of unlearning her pain.

The brain can cause a wide variety of mild to severe symptoms in virtually any area of the body. Cutting edge neuroscience research has given us a better understanding of how this happens. Timothy Noakes, an exercise physiologist, has studied how an athlete's brain reacts to running a marathon (Noakes, 2003). Dr. Noakes discovered why well-trained athletes "hit the wall" in endurance events: the pain and fatigue is due to their subconscious brain sounding an alarm warning them that they will run out of energy soon. Noakes explains that athletes must ignore these warning signals in order to finish the race, recognizing that there is no actual danger of physical harm. "Hitting the wall" is similar to the light on your car's gas gauge turning on to alert you that your gas is getting low; however, your car can still run fine for a while.

The subconscious brain is the driving force behind psychophysiologic reactions. The subconscious controls our bodily functions to protect us and help us adapt to our environment. Our reactions to our environment depend on both the innate and learned coding of our brain. Over our lifetime, our brains learn to respond to potentially dangerous situations. And, as Hebb famously noted, "when neurons fire together, they become wired together," and those neural pathways become more likely to fire the more they are activated (Hebb, 1949).

When I had low back pain several years ago, my back hurt every time I bent over. However, it turned out that my back was not actually damaged. It was my brain turning on pain because it predicted that I should have pain when I bent over. This new understanding led me to stop worrying about my back and remind myself that I was fine every time I bent over. In a few weeks, my back pain decreased and eventually went away. For more information on predictive coding, interoception, and how the brain constructs what we feel, see *How Emotions are Made* by Lisa Feldman Barrett (2017).

The Role of Stress in Childhood

It is not only current stress that can trigger painful reactions. Emotional experiences in childhood are imprinted in the brain. Several studies show that animals exposed in infancy to very stressful environments (such as separation from their mother or being exposed to painful stimuli) grow up to have overly active autonomic nervous system responses (McEwen, 1998; Arborelius and Eklund, 2007). Human infants who are exposed to repeated blood drawing within the first few weeks of life have increased pain when they have medical procedures several months later (Taddio, et. al., 2002). Adults who are exposed to traumatic events in childhood such as emotional, physical, or sexual abuse have a much greater chance of developing chronic pain (as well as anxiety and other psychological disturbances) (Anda, et. al., 2006). The emotional imprinting from early experiences is stored in the brain, and when a similar experience occurs later in life, the ANS reaction can start a painful process.

Researchers can measure markers of chronic stress, such as abnormalities in an ANS hormone, cortisol. One study found that adults who have abnormalities in cortisol production are more likely to develop chronic pain than those who do not have these abnormalities (McBeth, et. al., 2007). This further cements the powerful relationship between chronic stress and chronic pain.

How an Injury Can Start a Cycle of Pain

Sometimes the pain cycle is started by an injury, such as a strain, a sprain, or a fracture. When the injury occurs, the danger signals in the body and brain get fired. Usually these signals will decrease, and the pain will go away when the injury heals. Most acute injuries will heal within a few weeks. That is how long it usually takes for the body to repair any tissue breakdown that has occurred. After that, if the pain does not go away, there is something else going on. Many people are suffering from chronic pain that they believe is caused by an injury that occurred several months or years ago. That doesn't make sense, because fractures of even our biggest bones will heal in several weeks. The injury itself—whether from a sprain or a strain such as a whiplash injury—is not *causing* the pain. But an injury can trigger a series of events that lead to chronic pain. This point is quite often misunderstood, since many people have been told by doctors, physical therapists, or chiropractors that their injury never healed or set off misalignments that continue to cause pain. While I must avoid judging every single situation, I can say that in general, this concept is not supported by the research. Injuries to our body do heal. Even if there is scar tissue present, scar tissue doesn't cause pain. People with retained bullets or shrapnel or those who must walk with a limp due to an injury don't necessarily have pain.

Physical injuries are more likely to create chronic pain if there are stressful life circumstances occurring around the same time as the injury. If so, the pain signals set in motion by the injury can become learned, and a vicious cycle of pain may develop. The brain is always learning from the experiences that we have. When pain is triggered by a physical injury, the brain will need to "decide" whether to turn that pain off or continue to create it. That decision by the brain is made moment by moment depending on the inputs the brain is given. These inputs come from our past experiences as we have seen, our thoughts and emotions, and our reactions to the pain itself. As we shall see, the way that we react to the pain is a powerful determinant of whether the pain will resolve or become chronic. While we can't change our pasts, we can change how we respond to the pain itself and this is one way that we can train the brain to de-activate the neural circuits of pain.

Thoughts and Pain

A great deal of research has demonstrated how the brain actually controls pain. All pain has sensory, cognitive, and affective components (Wager, et. al., 2004). The **sensory** component includes descriptions of how pain is felt, such as aching, burning, sharpness, or numbing. The **cognitive** component is what you think about the pain: what the cause is, whether you believe it is temporary or permanent, controllable or curable. The **affective** component consists of your feelings and emotions about the pain, such as fear, worry, anger, and resentment. There are distinct areas of the nervous system that process these three components of pain (Melzack and Casey, 1968; Ploner et. al., 1999; Vogt and Sikes, 2000; Ochsner et. al., 2008). In order to eliminate chronic pain, all of the components need to be addressed. The ways in which people think about their pain and the feelings that are connected to it have great impact on the severity of the pain.

M.D. Lieberman and colleagues (2004) conducted a study in which people with irritable bowel syndrome were treated with a placebo pill. In those who responded with fewer symptoms (less pain, diarrhea, or constipation), they found that certain areas of the brain were activated while other areas were de-activated. In those whose symptoms did not decrease, they found opposite effects in the brain. This study demonstrates that what we think about our condition—the cognitive components of our pain—affects how our brain controls pain and other Mind Body Syndrome symptoms.

In a study published in the *Journal of the American Medical Association* (Waber, et. al., 2008), a group of researchers tested the pain responses of volunteers to a bracelet that gave gradated levels of electric shocks. All participants were first given a pill that they were told was a new medication similar to codeine, but faster acting. Half of the subjects were told that it cost about $2.50 per pill, while the others were told that each pill cost ten cents. Though all the pills were placebos, those who received the more "expensive" pills felt significantly less pain from the bracelet shocks than did those who were given the supposedly cheaper pills.

In a research study of people with chronic hand pain due to an ANS dysfunction condition known as complex regional pain syndrome (or reflex sympathetic dystrophy), subjects were shown pictures of hands in different positions. They were asked to imagine moving their hand into those positions. Results showed that they had increased pain and swelling of their hands just from imagining moving them (Moseley, et. al., 2008).

These studies demonstrate that what we think about pain can have a great impact on how we actually feel pain. Many studies also show how emotions affect how we experience pain.

Emotions and Pain

Several studies demonstrate the connection between emotions and pain. Mark Lumley and colleagues have published an excellent review of this topic (Lumley, et. al., 2011). There is a large overlap between Mind Body Syndrome and different types of anxiety disorders. More than a third of people with fibromyalgia or irritable bowel syndrome have high rates of post-traumatic stress disorder (PTSD) (Amir, et. al., 1997; Sherman, et. al., 2000). One study of a group of military veterans with PTSD showed 80 percent of them had chronic pain (Beckham, 1997). In a study of people with obsessive-compulsive disorder (OCD), situations that triggered their OCD symptoms were associated with an activated ACC in the brain (Fitzgerald, et. al., 2005).

John Burns (2008) studied pain thresholds in people with chronic low back pain. He found that when they recalled a time that had made them angry, they had increased activation of the lower back muscles and experienced more pain. They did not show increases in heart rate or blood pressure and did not have activation of muscle groups unrelated to the areas of pain, which shows that their bodies reacted to anger in a very specific area. In another study, volunteers were put in a situation that created either anxiety or anger and then instructed to either express their feelings normally, try to inhibit their feelings, or try not to show any feelings. After this they placed one hand in ice water. Those who were instructed not to feel or show anxiety or anger had less tolerance for the pain (Quartana and Burns, 2007). Finally, patients with low back pain were instructed to either suppress or not suppress anger during a stressful laboratory experiment. Those instructed to suppress their emotions reported more pain, both during and after the experiment (Burns, et. al., 2008). Together these studies show that both anxiety and anger can cause a lower pain threshold and can increase muscle tension. Suppression of emotions leads to even higher pain levels.

Brain imaging studies have also revealed the strong relationship between emotions and pain. For example, Eisenberger and her colleagues (2003 and 2006) have shown that when people are put in a laboratory situation where they are excluded or rejected by others, the brain's danger/alarm mechanism is activated and pain sensitivity is increased. The brain's danger signals are also activated by fear and worry (Fitzgerald, et. al., 2005; Das, et. al., 2005). Ethan Kross and colleagues performed separate brain scans in young adults who were given a mild physical pain and also shown a picture of an ex-lover who had broken up with them within the past six months (Kross, et. al., 2011). Not surprisingly, the same areas of the brain were activated by a physical injury and an emotional injury. Both physical pain and emotional pain are handled the same way in the brain and can cause real pain.

When pain develops, if we are unsure why it's there and our doctors are unable to explain it or make it go away, most people begin to worry about the pain and to fear that it will become a constant problem. These emotions then trigger pain circuits in the brain to become more pronounced, which, of course, tends to exacerbate the pain (Bailey, et. al., 2009; Asmundson and Katz, 2009). A vicious cycle of pain, fear of pain, decreased activity, and worry often ensues. When this happens, chronic pain becomes a way of life, and there is no way out of it until the thoughts and feelings which are driving the pain are addressed. As we shall see, this vicious cycle of pain leading to fear that leads to increases in pain is often the most important mechanism of the persistence of pain. The program in this book will teach you how to reverse this cycle in the brain to eliminate your pain or other MBS symptoms. For an excellent description of this phenomenon as seen in chronic back pain, see *Back Sense* (Siegel, et. al., 2001).

A unique study was conducted with a group of healthy volunteers and a group of people who had recovered from significant depression (Hooley, et. al., 2005). Both groups had brain MRIs taken while they listened to a tape recording of their own mothers, who had recorded thirty seconds of praise and also thirty seconds of criticism. Both groups had increases in activation of the "safety" mechanisms (an area of the brain known as the dorsolateral prefrontal cortext, DLPFC) when listening to the praise. When the healthy volunteers listened to the criticism, they also had increases in the DLPFC (demonstrating their resiliency to stress), but those with a history of depression had decreases in DLPFC activation, putting them at risk for developing pain. To summarize, when we experience difficult or stressful situations, especially if we have had significant stresses earlier in life and if we are unable to express or show how we feel, we will be at risk for our bodies to experience pain.

The Triggers of Pain

Once a pain cycle is initiated between the brain and the body, certain "triggers" will usually begin to develop and add to the painful responses. Most people have heard of the experiments of Ivan Pavlov, the Russian scientist, who rang a buzzer when he fed his dogs (Cunningham, 2001). He soon noticed the dogs would salivate when the buzzer rang, even if there was no food in sight. Their brains had learned that a buzzer meant food, so their bodies reacted accordingly. Several years ago, Robert Ader gave some mice cyclophosphamide, a powerful immune-suppressing medication, in a bowl with saccharine, which has a peculiar taste. Predictably, their immune systems became significantly suppressed. A few weeks later, after their immune systems recovered, he gave them a bowl with just saccharine. Their immune systems again became suppressed, demonstrating the power of triggers (Cohen, et. al., 1979). This study has been replicated in people as well (Goebel, et. al., 2002).

It is easy to see how certain triggers can develop in people with Mind Body Syndrome. Once a painful neural circuit (say, a headache) has started, if it occurs during a stressful situation that also happens to coincide with eating a certain food, or drinking red wine, or seeing a certain kind of light, or meeting a certain person, the brain will learn that association. Then the next time you are exposed to that chemical or situation, the headache can recur. This is the process of conditioning.

Foods are common triggers in abdominal and urinary tract conditions, such as irritable bowel syndrome, heartburn, bloating, as well as irritable bladder syndrome (interstitial cystitis), urinary frequency and pelvic pain. People with these conditions often find that certain foods aggravate their condition and many are told to avoid specific foods. Over time, more and more foods start to become triggers for these symptoms, leading to situations where people can eat only a limited range of foods and fear that they will be exposed to foods that will make them sick. The vast majority of the time, these are simply learned and conditioned responses, rather than actual allergies or direct effects of the foods themselves. The same process occurs to a more significant degree in the condition known as multiple chemical sensitivities. Physical activities can also be triggers. For example, someone with back pain will notice that walking, driving, sitting, or bending over will cause pain, and these actions will be associated with pain and become triggers for the pain. Over time, the pathways connecting these triggers to the pain will become stronger, and the pain cycle will become very well learned by the brain and the body.

Fortunately, these triggers can be overcome or, in psychological terms, extinguished, by unlearning this connection. The program in this book will teach you how to break these triggers that perpetuate pain and other Mind Body Syndrome symptoms.

Priming of Pain

Another important concept to understand is that of "priming." When we learn how to ride a bicycle or throw a ball, those neural circuits become engrained. Even if we haven't been on a bike or thrown a ball in several years, when we need to, those circuits will be activated, and we will perform that skill. Nerve impulses that are caused by a physical injury, such as a car accident or a fall, create a painful neural circuit between the brain and the body, which will typically diminish over a few days or weeks as the damaged body tissues heal. However, these neural circuits can lie dormant, and at some time in the future, if situations occur that create significant stress and emotional reactions, these pain pathways can re-emerge to create the same type of pain.

I evaluated a young woman with severe back pain. As a teenager, she had sustained a mild back injury from a fall during an athletic competition. Her injury healed, and she was fine for several years. However, when her fiancé broke off their engagement just prior to the wedding date, she developed back pain in the same area, although no new injury occurred. Her brain was primed to have back pain in that specific area, and it created pain in a place that was convenient since it had already been learned.

Dr. Lorimer Moseley is a leading pain researcher whose work is dedicated to understanding and explaining pain (see Butler and Moseley, *Explain Pain*, 2003 and Moseley, *Painful Yarns*, 2007). In *Painful Yarns*, he tells a story from his own life that helps us understand important mechanisms of pain. As a young boy, Lorimer took hikes in the country and frequently came home with lots of nicks and scrapes on his legs. Although his mother was often alarmed, they never bothered him or hurt him. While on a hike at age twenty-five, he got nicked on the leg and kept walking not thinking anything of it. When he got home, he saw the fang marks of the very poisonous Eastern Brown snake and found his left leg to be very swollen and painful. He spent several days in the hospital recovering from the bite and the left leg pain subsided. Five years later, he was walking in a park and noted a nick on his leg. He immediately fell to the ground experiencing a great deal of pain that was all the way up and down his left leg. He was rushed to the hospital only to find that he simply had a scrape, not a snake bite. Why all the pain? When he was a boy, his brain disregarded the mild pain from nicks and scrapes because they were interpreted as "not dangerous" and simply part of the enjoyment of walking in the country. However, after the life-threatening situation with the snakebite, his brain now interpreted a small scrape as "very dangerous" and activated the same pain pathways that were learned five years earlier.

What is amazing is that the pain after a small scrape on Lorimer's leg lasted for two weeks. He's a pain researcher; he understands pain; he knew that nerve pathways rather than tissue damage caused his whole leg to feel real pain; yet the pain persisted for two weeks! The nerve patterns were activated and took a while to calm down and reverse, which they eventually did. But what might have happened if he didn't understand pain, and after one week he went to his doctor and asked, 'Why am I still having so much pain from a small scrape? The doctor might say, "Oh, I'm afraid that you might have "post-snake bite venom" syndrome. It's a chronic disorder. We don't know what causes it and we have no effective treatment for it." This is exactly the situation that occurs to people with fibromyalgia, whiplash, and chronic fatigue syndrome. The labeling of these disorders as being chronic and incurable leads to more fear, more resentment, and more pain. Another factor can greatly activate pain pathways. What if, during those two weeks after the scrape, something was happening in Lorimer's life: maybe his son got arrested, his mother passed away, or his wife had an affair. Emotions associated with those events trigger the same brain pathways that activate pain thus turning what would have been a self-limited disorder into a chronic one with little hope of cure.

It is very easy to think of pain as an enemy. It can hurt so much that it may be impossible to imagine how the mind could be powerful enough to produce it, or why the mind would do that to its own body! Pain can feel like our mind is betraying us for no good reason. But consider how the brain responds to inputs. When you touch a hot stove, the signals from the fingers go up to the brain and the brain sends a "danger" message. The brain determines how much pain is produced in response to how much danger it perceives. The more perceived danger, the more pain. Larger injuries and those that are in sensitive areas (such as the fingers, face, eyes and head) tend to produce more pain. Even in the case of physical injury, the brain determines how much pain will be manufactured, or even if pain will occur at all!

Pain is a protective mechanism. We need pain! In fact, children who are born without the ability to feel pain due to a genetic disorder often have severe problems as they frequently get injuries without knowing it.

A friend of mine told me about a man he saw diving in the ocean for conch shells. When he emerged with the conch shell, he showed it to his wife on the beach and was beaming. He had no pain until he noticed that his legs were bleeding due to cuts from the coral reef. A construction worker in Britain jumped off scaffolding and landed on a large exposed nail, which pierced his work boot. He immediately began screaming in pain and was rushed to the hospital. Pain and sedation medications given through an IV were necessary to try to lessen his pain. When doctors removed the boot, they found that the nail was lodged between two toes and had not injured him at all (Fisher, et. al., 1995). In both of these cases, the brain controlled if and how much pain occurred, while the amount of physical injury was a secondary factor.

Our brains were designed to alert us to danger. When the pain circuits in the brain are activated, we feel pain; when we have a sudden scare, we feel afraid. In both situations, our brain is trying to alert us to physical or emotional danger to protect us from threats to our health and well being. It is telling us to get help, pay attention, or wake up. In the case of mind body pain, anxiety, or depression, your brain is letting you know you are in some kind of danger, and so it activates very powerful neural circuits. It is not really known why the brain would create physical pain due to stressful life situations. As I have mentioned, we know that a physical injury and an emotional injury activate the very same painful neural circuits in the brain, so that the pain due to an emotional injury is exactly the same as the pain from a physical injury, i.e., real pain! All pain is real and all pain is actually generated by the brain.

Why would the brain create physical pain due to stressful situations? One theory that I find compelling is that the human species survived and thrived due to banding together in clans and groups. Since survival depended on being in the group, getting kicked out of the group or being ostracized could be a kind of a death sentence. Therefore, doing something against the group, such as beating up someone or challenging someone of authority, could result in being shamed or ridiculed or expelled. This process may have linked emotional injuries to severe consequences and therefore the brain adapted to this situation by sending out powerful warning messages of danger. This is a just a theory, of course. We don't really know why physical pain and many other symptoms can occur in the absence of a physical injury, but we do know that it does happen on a regular basis in all of us. Our brain is just trying to help us by alerting us to some kind of danger. It is our task to figure out what the danger is, or if there is really any danger at all!

Another fascinating topic that comes up is why does the brain choose to create pain in a specific area versus another area in the body. The short answer is that we don't know. The subconscious brain has the capacity to produce a wide variety of pain and other symptoms as we have seen. However, there are times when the location of the pain seems to make some sense. Here are some examples of "reasons" why certain pains may occur.

1. Symbolic — pain in the neck can mean someone is a pain in your neck; stomach upset can mean there is something in your life that "makes you sick," or foot pain can mean there is something that "you can't stand."

2. Contagious — symptoms are often contagious from person to person or on a society level. This is probably what is happening, at least to some degree, with so-called "long COVID" syndrome. There is widespread awareness of this syndrome in society at large and the brain can easily pick up on those symptoms.

3. Injury — pain can occur at the spot of an old injury that has already healed as the brain has easily built in neural circuits for that pain.

4. Familial — certain symptoms run in families, so the brain might simply choose one of those, such as headaches, back pain, etc.

5. Mechanical — the brain may choose an area where the person is using that part of the body quite a bit, such as hands with typing, back with manual labor, or eyes with computer use.

I treated a man who had a recurrence of MBS symptoms of pain and anxiety as he was buying a new home. I explained to him that his brain was interpreting this act as if he were running into a burning building. Our job is to learn how to recognize these symptoms as primitive warning signals. As with a fire alarm, we are thankful that it alerted us. However, if it's a false alarm and there is no fire, we simply turn the alarm off and reset it. That is exactly what we need to do for Mind Body Syndrome: understand that there is no real physical danger, thank the brain for alerting us, investigate our lives for the source of the message our brain is sending, and turn off the alarm. The program in this book is designed to teach you to do all of that.

chapter 4

How Pain Develops: The Role of the Mind

We must never take a person's testimony, however sincere, that he has felt nothing, as proof positive that no feeling has been there. — William James

The Psychological Basis for Mind Body Syndrome

Many people have trouble accepting that severe pain and other dramatic symptoms can be caused wholly by the interaction between the mind and the body. Not only is it true, it is common. Bodily reactions to mental events occur in most people on a regular basis—we just don't notice them, or we attribute them to purely physical causes. The truth is that the body is a barometer of the mind, and it reflects what is going on in the mind every minute of every day. Once you are aware of this connection, you will see the signs in yourself and your family and friends on a regular basis.

After I gave a lecture a few years ago, a physician approached me and told me his story. While in the Vietnam War, he was hit with shrapnel in one leg, after his unit came under attack and several of his buddies were also injured or killed. He was medevacked out of the battle field. He regained full function of his leg, was pain-free, became a doctor and had a wonderful family. Occasionally, "out of the blue," he would start to limp and have leg pain (in the same area of the original pain) that would last for a few minutes and then go away. He had no idea why, but it recurred every year or two. One day, a few years ago, during an episode of leg pain and limping, his wife said to him, "Do you hear that helicopter?" He replied, "No, I didn't, but I hear it now." And the next time he began limping, there was a helicopter overhead. As soon as he recognized that the sound of a helicopter triggered his limping, the limping vanished. At a subconscious level in his brain, the sound reminded him of his traumatic experiences during the war and caused his brain to activate a learned neural circuit, without him even being aware of the sound that had triggered his physical reaction.

A Brief History of Mind Body Syndrome

To help understand how MBS develops, let's first look at the history of how psychological mechanisms have caused disorders now recognizable as MBS. In the 1600s through the 1800s, a common response to significant stress was paralysis in a limb. This sudden inability to use an arm or leg was not due to tissue disease, stroke, or damage to the nervous system. In those days, this type of paralysis was viewed as a common medical condition, rather than as a physical manifestation of psychological distress. In modern times, we call this a conversion disorder because there is no pathology in the brain or body—yet the affected person cannot move the "paralyzed" arm or leg.

In the 1930s, a physician reported on the case of a young nun who left the convent and secretly married without her parents' knowledge. As she sat down to write her parents a letter about what she had done, she could not move her arm. Later that day, she went to church for confession and suddenly was unable to speak. This was clearly a case of significant symptoms being caused by the subconscious mind. Though she may not have felt extremely distressed, her subconscious mind acted to prevent her from revealing the marriage either verbally or in writing—probably because of significant fear and/or guilt (Harriman, 1935).

An important advance in medicine was the discovery of deep tendon reflexes. The simple test of striking a tendon with a reflex hammer can quickly distinguish pathological from psychological paralysis. Amazingly, once doctors could do this test, the number of people with this type of conversion disorder decreased substantially, and now the condition is rare. When doctors and the general public come to view a medical condition as psychologically induced, it is less likely to occur. See *From Paralysis to Fatigue* for an excellent discussion of this phenomena (Shorter, 1992).

Even though we see fewer cases of conversion disorder than in the past, this disorder still occurs somewhat regularly. There are singers who may suddenly become unable to sing on stage. It is well documented cultures that people in certain small groups can have very unusual reactions, such as wild thrashing about, falling asleep for days on end, developing muscle spasms or many other symptoms, that become contagious within that group (O'Sullivan, 2021). There is even a series of children who have fallen victim to a type of catatonia where they are unable to move, open their eyes, or even eat for months or years on end (Nunn, 2014). In all of these cases, there is absolutely nothing physically wrong with them. For various reasons, their subconscious brain has taken over their body and created these very odd and serious symptoms. Please know that these symptoms are real, very real and very powerful. These folks are not faking or imagining these symptoms, they are unable to stop them voluntarily. These cases demonstrate the power of the brain over us. If the brain can cause these symptoms, it can certainly cause headaches, back pain, fatigue or insomnia.

Choices of the Mind

The subconscious mind is unlikely to produce symptoms that will be easily seen as psychological. But since humans continue to experience great stresses and strong emotions, paralysis has been replaced by chronic back pain, fibromyalgia, fatigue, irritable bowel syndrome, and many other symptoms (Shorter, 1992).

Most medical students have seen that some of their classmates will tend to get certain symptoms when they learn about them in school. This type of suggestibility is a form of what's known as social contagion. Nicholas Christakis and James Fowler have studied social contagion and found that smoking, obesity, and happiness are all at least partially determined by contact with people whom we see socially or at work (Christakis and Fowler, 2008; Christakis and Fowler, 2007; Fowler and Christakis, 2008). In Germany, surveys of the prevalence of back pain were done for several years in both East and West Germany, beginning with the fall of the Berlin Wall and the reunification of Germany (Raspe, et. al., 2008). The levels of back pain were much lower in East Germany prior to reunification, but these levels rose to meet the levels of back pain in West Germany after the two countries merged. The authors gave this reason: "We hypothesize that back pain is a communicable disease and suggest a harmful influence of back-related beliefs and attitudes transmitted from West to East Germany via mass media and personal contacts." We are bombarded with television ads for medications for restless leg syndrome, fibromyalgia, migraine headaches, and insomnia—all of which are typically forms of MBS. These ads actually increase the number of people who get these conditions, because the subconscious mind will be more likely to create and perpetuate these common symptoms when stressful situations occur in life.

The symptoms that occur when we are under significant stress can vary greatly. I saw a teenager who developed a variety of symptoms over the course of a year. I was certain these symptoms were all caused by MBS, because extensive medical testing showed no tissue breakdown disorders and he recovered fully with MBS treatment. He was going through a significant amount of family stress and developed hip pain, then headaches, then chest pain, then fainting spells, then stomach pains, then the headaches again, then leg pains. All these symptoms were caused by the subconscious mind creating physical symptoms in response to his stressful situation. Interestingly, he never developed any signs of anxiety or depression, which are common in adults with MBS. This would have been less acceptable to him as a young male, so his mind "chose" other pathways to express the tension.

A few years ago, I saw a young man who had developed severe pain. His sister had died suddenly, and during the mourning period he was invited to a bachelor's party for a friend. He didn't think he should attend, but his friends convinced him to go. At the party, there was a lot of drinking and nudity, and he received an erotic massage. The next morning he woke up with pain in his groin. He went to many different doctors—including urologists, neurologists, pain doctors, and anesthesiologists—and even a nationally renowned medical center. Each doctor heard the same story, "I just woke up with this pain one day," and none asked about the context of his life. He was treated with many different medications, painkillers, injections, and nerve blocks—to no avail. But it's pretty obvious that the cause for his pain was his conflicted feelings about going to the party. The groin pain was a manifestation of guilt. This is a good example of the theory that strong emotions are often too dangerous or disturbing to be felt or expressed and therefore these emotions are kept in the subconscious by means of suppression. The resultant tension in the mind is expressed as pain or other MBS symptoms as a distraction or a warning from these strong subconscious emotions (Sarno, 2006). After three painful years, the young man finally sought treatment for Mind Body Syndrome and became pain free.

This story illustrates a common situation that seems obvious when understanding that the brain can control our body. But many other circumstances are not so easily apparent as being due to a significant stressful state. A more common situation is that an individual notices the gradual onset of headaches, back pain, abdominal or pelvic pain, loose stool, frequent urination, ringing in the ears, trouble sleeping or other common symptoms and there is no major life stressor going on that of which they are aware. They may have stress in their lives, but doesn't everyone? Of course we do. Sometimes the stress that is causing the mind body symptoms is just "life" and the everyday stresses of work, family, neighbors and making ends meet. In fact, most people get some kinds of mild mind body symptoms at times, just by being human. Another common occurrence is that after an injury happens, the pain due to that injury just doesn't go away. This common scenario is usually due to a combination of life stressors and often a persistent worry about the injury or the pain of the injury that activates the ongoing neural circuits of pain or other symptoms.

The Subconscious Mind

Many studies document the role of the subconscious mind in determining human behavior. It is estimated that approximately 95 percent of our thoughts, feelings, and memories reside in the subconscious (Wilson, 2002). While a human brain can take in about eleven million bits of information each second, the conscious brain can process only about forty bits. We are responding each moment to a huge amount of information being poured into our subconscious minds (Wilson, 2002).

Most of our daily actions are guided by our subconscious mind. We learn how to do routine things, and these actions become automatic—how we chew and swallow, how we walk, speak, drive a car, throw a baseball. We don't consciously think about how to do these things, we just do them. As described in *Strangers to Ourselves: Discovering the Adaptive Unconscious* by Timothy Wilson (2002) and by Daniel Wegner in *The Illusion of Conscious Will* (2002), these routine actions are all produced by learned neurological patterns in the subconscious part of the brain.

What about thoughts and actions that are not so commonly performed? What about things that we decide to do, such as which clothes to wear, what to order at a restaurant, whom to ask for a date? These acts too are controlled to a great degree by the subconscious mind. As described by Wegner, we are not consciously aware of most actions until we perform them. Even the simplest act of lifting a finger has been shown to have a subconscious component that occurs in the brain before we are aware that we have decided to lift the finger (Wegner, 2002).

Many research studies show that our subconscious mind drives our reactions to everyday situations. In one study, people subliminally presented with words such as "old," "wise," "retired," and "gray" walked more slowly from the room than a control group who were presented with random words (Bargh, et. al., 1996). People who were shown aggressive words in a subliminal fashion interpreted behavior of others as being more hostile (Bargh and Pietromonaco, 1982), and those who were shown subliminal words related to assertiveness were more likely to interrupt the investigator than those who were shown subliminal words related to politeness (Bargh, 1990). People who briefly held an iced coffee drink in their hand rated a stranger as being less friendly than did people who held a warm cup of coffee (Williams and Bargh, 2008).

Reactions to Stress

As we grow up, we are exposed to certain stressful events, and the emotional memories associated with these events are stored in the amygdala, hippocampus and other brain structures. When physical stress occurs, such as an injury or accident, our body responds instantly to protect ourselves by activation of the danger/alarm mechanism. The same danger mechanism is also activated by social stress that triggers emotional reactions. The danger mechanism responds so fast that we do not become aware of most emotions until we actually notice the reactions in our body, such as trembling, increased heart rate, or sweating. This is so we can react swiftly to danger by fleeing, fighting, freezing, or submitting.

The standard view of the sequence of events that causes emotions used to be: when you see a bear, you feel afraid, and then you run. However, more than 100 years ago, psychologist William James explained that actually we run first and then we feel fear (James, 1884). Joseph Ledoux, in *The Emotional Brain* (1996), points out that the neural circuits that sense a dangerous situation will send signals to the amygdala within twelve milliseconds. It takes twice as long for the signals to get to the conscious part of the brain (LeDoux, 1996). I often refer to this rapid process as "emotional speed dial," because our bodies can typically react to emotional triggers before we are even aware of the trigger. The brain has been shown to respond to visual and other stimuli that are presented at a subconscious level and these stimuli can cause pain and other reactions in our bodies (Whalen, 1998; Knight, et. al., 2003).

Stored forever in our brains, emotional memories can trigger physical or emotional responses. I had a patient who as a child lived with an abusive aunt and uncle during the week and stayed with his loving and kind mother on the weekends. When he was married and in his thirties, he noticed that he would get very depressed if his wife worked an evening shift on Sunday, but not if she worked on any other evening. He didn't understand why until we reviewed his history, and then it became clear that the emotional memory he had of leaving his mother on Sundays to return to the abusive aunt and uncle was causing the reaction. Ohman and colleagues showed that fears can be induced without our conscious awareness and that, many years later, we can react to an object or a situation without being aware of the emotions causing the reaction (Ohman, 1992; LeDoux, 1996).

I saw a young woman with low back pain that was clearly not due to a structural problem based upon the evidence from her history and her imaging studies. She had had a recurrence of pain twice in the last two years, both times during the month of May. Her father happened to be in the room with her when I asked both of them if they recall any significant events that happened to them during the month of May. They both initially said "no, nothing at all." I chose to just wait a minute to see if they thought of something that might be significant. I watched silently as a tear rolled down the cheek of the teen-ager and then a tear also appeared in her father's eye. Her sister had suddenly passed away during the month of May a couple of years earlier. Her brain was responding to the anniversary of her passing without her conscious awareness.

Messages from the Subconscious

In our modern lives, we rarely encounter predators. However, our brains are designed to constantly scan our environment for any signs of danger. When we have significant stresses that remind us of something that caused fear, anger, or guilt earlier in life, our mind will interpret these as dangers. In these situations, our subconscious mind will try to alert us to a problem or protect us from something it perceives as harmful. Unfortunately, our brains do not use words to tell us that there is a perceived danger. Our bodies just react, often with pain. When we are faced with very stressful situations, especially when we feel trapped and unable to find a solution, our brains react as if we are in grave danger. The brain will activate the danger/alarm mechanism, and it can cause tension in certain specific muscles—tension that creates real pain. Over time, the pain can worsen or become widespread. I often use this metaphor to describe this process: "Your body was knocking to let you know that something was bothering you. But you didn't understand it. So, it knocked louder and louder, by creating more pain or new symptoms. When you didn't listen, it rang the doorbell, and finally it threw a rock through a window to get your attention."

An important predictor of whether someone will have successful back surgery is job satisfaction (Gatchel, et. al., 1995). Back pain will often develop in people who are experiencing severe difficulties in their jobs but cannot quit them. Their subconscious mind will often try to "protect" them by causing pain to get them out of the distressing situation. For example, one study found that women who experienced high workloads, little control, and "bullying" in the workplace were more likely to develop fibromyalgia (Kivimaki, et. al., 2004). In the case of Vickie, the woman in chapter 2 with severe headaches, the pain was her body's way of trying to protect her by causing her to leave her job. Despite treatments by many doctors, her headaches lasted for seventeen years until she sought help from this program.

BARRY WAS A THIRTY-FIVE-YEAR-OLD MAN *who had a significant accident while on the job as a firefighter. He was bruised and shaken up, but the doctors found no broken bones when he was seen in the emergency room. The next day, he developed neck pain, and this pain just didn't go away. He had an MRI that showed only mild abnormalities, and his doctors suggested physical therapy. However, that didn't help, and he had to go on disability because he could not work with such severe pain. Over time, he took pain medications and tried to exercise, but nothing helped. After nine months on disability, he came to see me. Barry told me that he had had similar injuries in the past but had always bounced back and had been back at work within a few weeks. It didn't appear that this injury was much different from his other injuries. When I asked if there was something else that might have been different in this situation, he told me that one of his friends had died in the fire. After examining him and finding no evidence of nerve damage in his neck or arms, I explained that he did not have tissue damage in his neck but that the pain was caused by Mind Body Syndrome. I explained that consciously he wanted to return to work but that his nervous system had become sensitized as subconsciously he had feelings of fear, anger, and guilt caused by his friend's death. Barry's pain was real but also curable. He realized that he could get better and started doing the exercises recommended in this book. In three weeks, his pain was 80 percent better. By six weeks, he was back at work.*

The subconscious mind can choose which symptoms occur during times of stress. That is why people who grow up with a parent with headaches will often develop headaches. Someone who grows up with relatives with abdominal pain or back pain will often develop those symptoms decades later. As noted earlier, social contagion is a mechanism by which specific symptoms can be triggered.

Sometimes the way our bodies react can give us a clue to what the mind is trying to tell us.

The pain can occur in an appropriate spot—such as the groin pain in the young man after the bachelor's party. When someone develops a pain in the buttocks, there may be someone in their lives who is a "pain in the butt." Someone who develops difficulty swallowing may be reacting to a situation in life that is "hard to swallow." I evaluated a woman with pain in the bottom of her feet. While waiting in line one day, she realized there was a situation in her life that she "just couldn't stand anymore." People often develop headaches before appointments or social situations that are likely to be stressful or where there are people that they have strong feelings about. Often they will be unaware of those strong feelings; they will be subconscious feelings. In fact, emotions are more likely to cause reactions in our bodies when we are unaware that they are influencing us (LeDoux, 1996).

This process occurs on a regular, probably daily, basis in all of us. Our brains constantly monitor our environment for any potential situations that may be stressful or "dangerous." These occur almost every day and the mild stresses of finding a parking space, being late for a meeting, having to have a difficult conversation, worrying about a child, or getting sick are processed in our brains and evaluated. When the brain feels that one of these situations is sufficiently dangerous, even if we are obviously not in real danger, the brain may send a small message of alarm. We may get a slight tingling in our hand or foot, a slight stomach upset, a sudden buzzing noise in the ears, a tightness in the chest, or a deep sigh. These sensations typically last only a few seconds or minutes. Most of the time, we don't pay much attention to these sensations and are unaware that we are even thinking about something worrisome, as those thoughts and feelings are subconscious.

As mentioned in the last chapter, prior learning or priming is also a way in which the subconscious mind chooses a particular symptom. Someone who has injured a certain area is more likely to develop MBS pain in that area because the neurological pattern of pain and has already been established, and the brain remembers it.

I developed pain shooting down my left arm many years ago during a stressful situation. The pain eventually subsided, but when I get stressed it can reappear for short periods. My brain has not forgotten how to create this particular pain. Now I know what causes it, however, and I can get it to go away by recognizing that I may be stressed about something, dealing with the stress as best I can, and gently letting my subconscious mind know that I don't need the pain to alert me to a dangerous situation or get me out of something that I don't want to do. Or, upon reflection, there is really nothing specifically stressful going on in my life at the time. It may be the brain's danger signals just got activated out of habit or just falling back into a default circuit or due to some trigger that I'm not really aware of. Then I can just smile and calmly move on with what I'm doing so that my brain knows nothing is wrong and it will allow that circuit to turn off in a few minutes or so.

Components of the Subconscious Mind

Sigmund Freud was one of the most influential thinkers of the twentieth century. Although several scientists recognized that there was a subconscious part of the mind as early as the mid-1800s (Wilson, 2002), Freud helped us understand many more things about the subconscious. In particular, it has now been conclusively shown that Freud was correct when he proposed these tenets of modern psychology: childhood experiences have powerful effects on personality and later social relationships; we are not aware of most of our thoughts and emotions (they are subconscious); we commonly have conflicting feelings that occur at the same time towards certain individuals or situations; and we frequently act and react to people and situations through subconscious mechanisms (Westen, 1999). Of course, we are now well aware that many of Freud's ideas were wrong and sometimes dangerously so. Please do not think that I am unaware of this or that I take all of Freud's writings as gospel (Bornstein, 2005).

Neuroscientists have now confirmed that the subconscious mind is the major driving force behind almost everything we do on a daily basis. The subconscious mind causes most of us to have mild physical and psychological symptoms on a regular basis, and it can cause some of us to have chronic and serious pain and debilitating symptoms.

There is a useful way to think about how our minds work and what are the elements that make us "tick." There is a strong need to feel safe and protected, to feel connected to those who care about us, and to feel loved and needed. On the other hand, there is also a strong need to become independent, to be assertive of our wants and needs, and to be able to make decisions that affect our lives. Children who grow up with these needs being met are likely to be able to trust others, be loving and kind to themselves and others, and develop strong relationships. Their brain will tend to feel safe, even when there is stress or conflicts. They are less likely to develop MBS, although as we have mentioned, everyone can develop some mind body symptoms at times. However, children who grow up in situations that are stressful or traumatic, or if they were overly criticized, or were neglected in some ways, or were exposed to physical, sexual or emotional abuse, are more likely to feel unsafe during their whole lives. They are more likely to be harsh with themselves, put themselves last, to feel guilty, and to let others dictate how they live. They are more likely to be fearful and resentful. These feelings can have profound impacts that make MBS more likely, in childhood or at any time later in life.

The Impact of Childhood Hurts

As just mentioned, some children suffer severely from neglect, physical abuse, sexual abuse, or emotional abuse. But every child, even if not overtly abused, gets hurt in some ways. When parents get divorced or argue, when parents are critical or withhold love or give only conditional love, these actions produce pain for their children. Similar reactions can occur in response to taunting or teasing by siblings or other children. One of the most common statements I hear when I evaluate patients is "I never felt loved by my parents," or "I often felt that my father (or mother) would love me only if I acted in certain ways."

Many studies show that childhood hurts lead to an overly sensitive autonomic nervous system in adulthood. In mice, dogs, and monkeys, stressful experiences at an early age cause hyperactivity of the autonomic nervous system, leading to an exaggerated fight, flight, or freeze response (McEwen, 1998). Someone with an overactive autonomic nervous system is more likely to develop Mind Body Syndrome.

Childhood hurts will be remembered in the brain, and these emotional memories can be easily and rapidly triggered (on "speed dial") by similar experiences in adults. I saw a man who had a very difficult childhood due to a parental divorce and a father who never took time for him and never showed love for him. When the boy was twelve, his father remarried and sent him to live at a youth home, where he spent the rest of his adolescence. Despite this adversity, he became quite resilient as an adult, found work, and eventually married and had children. He had almost no contact with his father for many years. One day he asked his father, who was visiting the area, to stop by and see his grandchildren. His father came by in a drunken state, stayed only a few minutes, and left. Within a few days, the son developed severe stomach pains, back pain, and anxiety. For years, he sought medical care, never got a clear diagnosis, and ended up taking many different medications without relief. When we met, I told him: "Your father had poured the gasoline for all those years of your childhood, and when you asked him to do something for your children, he lit a match which ignited all the anger and resentment that had built up in your emotional memory. You could handle him neglecting and abusing you, but when he did a similar thing to your children, you had so many strong subconscious feelings that it erupted in your body." In fact, whenever he drank any alcohol after his father's visit, he got violently ill. For those who have had significant traumas in childhood, such as physical, emotional, or sexual abuse; abandonment; bullying; or other obvious difficulties, it is usually easy to identify the relationship between childhood issues and stressors later in life that trigger MBS symptoms.

Often the events that create the emotional priming in childhood are subtle. Fortunately, most people were not exposed to significant emotional, physical, or sexual abuse. In general, those with the greatest number of MBS syndromes are those who have had more significant childhood issues are more likely to have personality traits of guilt, self-criticism, low self-esteem, high expectations for self, extreme responsibility for others, and self-sacrifice. However, most people have had some form of MBS symptoms occur in their lifetime. Those with less obvious childhood stressors and people who describe their childhood as happy also get MBS. That occurs because everyone gets some form of MBS at some point in their lives, whether the resulting symptoms are mild, moderate or severe. It is part of the human condition.

A team of researchers has conducted studies on children whose parents offer love only on a conditional basis. These studies found that people who grow up with parents who give attention and affection only if certain tasks (such as educational or sports achievement, or specific behaviors) are performed were more likely to have low self-esteem, more self-criticism and guilt, and a conflicted relationship with their parents (Assor, et. al., 2004; Roth, et. al., 2009).

Even mild degrees of low self-esteem and the perception of not being good enough can be enough to trigger MBS symptoms. I saw a man who had a sudden onset of severe tinnitus (ringing in the ears) when he was fifty-two years old. He had no history of childhood abuse or neglect and had loving parents. The only childhood hurt we identified was when he moved from a lower-class neighborhood at age ten to a middle-class neighborhood. He was overweight, wore the "wrong" clothes, and got teased by the kids at his new school, which caused him to feel inadequate and embarrassed. He had no symptoms at all until he was twenty-seven years old, when he had an anxiety attack while working at a church on a project. He was a new member of this church, which he felt to be more prestigious than his old church. He was trying to fit in and be accepted. Years later, at age fifty-two, his ears started ringing just days before Thanksgiving, a day when he and his wife always went to her mother's house for dinner. He told me that his mother-in-law "never liked me, never accepted me, never thought I was good enough for her daughter." It became clear that his symptoms were a reactivation of a subtle childhood hurt—not being accepted in his new neighborhood—that had lived in his emotional memory for all those years.

Careful questioning and evaluation will almost always lead to a clear understanding of the causes of MBS, if you pay close attention to childhood events and how those can get triggered in adolescence or adulthood. I have interviewed hundreds of people with MBS and, so far, there have been only a handful of people for whom the source of their symptoms did not become clear to both me and the patient after an in-depth interview.

Having said that, there are some people for whom there is no obvious life stressor occurring at the time of onset of MBS. Sometimes, the stressor is an injury or an accident or an illness. It is necessary for the brain's danger signal to become activated when one gets sick or hurt. For example, we now know that when you catch a cold or the flu, the danger signal will activate feelings of fatigue to encourage you to rest and recuperate. Since most illnesses are short-term and all injuries will heal over time, the brain's danger signal will usually turn off and not generate MBS. But if there is significant fear or worry about the injury or the illness, the brain may generate ongoing symptoms of MBS. Although all of the data isn't in yet, this appears to be occurring to a significant number of people with long haul COVID (Paul, 2022; Matta, 2022) and a host of other disorders that are beginning to appear to be manifestations of MBS, such as chronic Lyme disease, mast cell activation syndrome, chronic Epstein-Barr virus (EBV), mild Ehlers-Danlos syndrome, and others.

The Role of Conscience

The conscience within the subconscious mind expects us to perform our obligations and duties. This part of the mind is the seat of guilt, shame, humiliation, self-criticism, self-blame, the need to be liked, the need to be good, high self-expectations, low self-esteem, and perfectionism. Those who grew up with a strong conscience are less likely to speak up for themselves and assert themselves. They are more likely to do many things for others and neglect doing things for themselves. They are often people who are shy and reserved, who don't like to draw attention to themselves, and who tend to hold emotions in. People with MBS almost always have many of these characteristics and emotions. Some families, some cultures, and even some religions teach children to emphasize these characteristics early in life. Many of my patients grew up in religions that tend to emphasize guilt and self-criticism. I rarely see people who are selfish and narcissistic in this program. Rather, it is the "good and kind" people of the world who tend to suffer with Mind Body Syndrome.

The subconscious mind is likely to produce physical symptoms at times of severe stress as an escape mechanism for the buildup of emotions that have no other outlet. A woman developed back pain when she was called on to care for her ailing mother, who had always been demanding and critical of her. Her conflict was between the moral obligation she felt to her mother and the anger and resentment toward her that started in childhood. She also felt guilty about resenting the work she had to do for her mother. She felt trapped, and that created tremendous tension in the mind. For her and many of my patients, the mind is like a pressure cooker, and there is often no outlet for these strong feelings. In the face of this tremendous conflict within the mind, the conscience will often not even allow these feelings to come into consciousness. These strong subconscious feelings were perceived by the brain as danger signals that were expressed as back pain.

In addition to earlier emotional events and the presence of personality traits of guilt, self-criticism, or needing to please, a third key element in the development of MBS is perceived (and often real) powerlessness. Most of the time when MBS symptoms develop, there is a feeling of being trapped in some way. It may be that one is trapped in a job with a very difficult boss or backbiting colleagues. Or it may be that one feels trapped with an injury that doesn't appear to have healed or an illness that causes a great deal of fear and worry. I saw a woman who felt trapped in a difficult marriage who had severe knee pain for a year. When the marriage was finally dissolved, her knee pain disappeared. Another way to be trapped is to be unable to express one's deep feelings. I think of this as being "verbally" trapped, when there are no close friends or relatives to whom one can disclose emotions. Many times, the emotions and situations causing MBS symptoms are so shameful or unacceptable or trigger so much guilt that the feelings are kept hidden by the subconscious mind. Those who feel trapped and tend to be unable to speak up for themselves are likely to suppress feelings of anger or resentment.

Any of these strong feelings and conflicts within the mind can easily create physical symptoms. I recently worked with a woman who had severe fibromyalgia pain that disappeared after taking this program. When I asked her the most important thing that she did to help herself, she told me that she had learned to fully express her emotions (for the first time in her life), and finally decided to stand up for herself, to not let everyone "walk all over her," and to make some decisions to do things she wanted to do, rather than continually accede to others' desires.

The Role of Gender

Women are more likely than men to have MBS. Many more women than men have migraine headaches, TMJ joint pain, and fibromyalgia, and women have slightly more back pain. The reason has eluded explanation for many years. If one understands how MBS develops, it appears that there are several potential explanations. First, women are more likely to be socialized to be deferential and take care of the needs of others before attending to their own needs. They are also more likely to be the victims of abuse. Women are more often in employment positions that are subservient and at the same time are expected to manage most of the duties in the home. They are also more likely to be in situations where they are caring for children, for aging parents, or for grandparents.

Women are more likely to be oriented toward wanting to please others and feel like they should be better or do more, and they are less likely to assert themselves. Men are more likely to be assertive and blame others rather than themselves for problems in their lives. In fact, two very large studies of men and women around the world showed that women are more likely to be conscientious and agreeable, and to worry. Surprisingly, these differences are greater in North America and Europe than in countries with more traditional cultures (Costa, et. al., 2001; Schmitt et. al., 2008).

Obviously, men also get MBS, and many men have endured childhood hurts and have very strong feelings of obligation and guilt and other indications of a highly developed conscience. In fact, each of our bodies is a barometer of what is going on in our environment and how we react to it. The events in our early lives condition us. If we've been hurt on a regular basis, an adaptive reaction would be to learn to please others to try to gain favor or to avoid others to avoid getting hurt. But there is often a cost to these reactions. When we experience stressful events that trigger deep emotions of suppressed anger, guilt, fear, or sadness, our bodies will often warn us of the situation by producing pain, anxiety, depression, insomnia, or fatigue. One thing that I often tell people is that the reason that they have Mind Body Syndrome is not that they are weak or crazy or incompetent—it is because they are human. Because of how we are constructed, the interaction between the mind and body frequently causes the body to react to thoughts and feelings.

Mind Body Syndrome and Health Care

In 1976, the social critic Ivan Illich warned of the potential iatrogenic consequences of labeling diseases: that the medical profession can actually make people sick (Illich, 1976). When patients with MBS are labeled as having degenerative disc disease on the basis of an MRI or as having fibromyalgia because they have widespread body pain, symptoms can be exacerbated and patients harmed by medical diagnoses. This occurs because the diagnosis creates fear and the belief that there is something seriously wrong with one's body. These emotions activate the danger/alarm mechanism, which creates even more pain by ramping up the learned neural circuits of MBS.

Yet there is also danger in certain diagnoses often given by some "alternative" medical practitioners, such as chronic yeast infection and adrenal fatigue. Such diagnoses can have effects similar to traditional medical labeling, turning a person with MBS symptoms that are due to stress and emotions into a patient with a condition that needs to be treated by herbal remedies or other interventions.

Most people have physical and psychological symptoms on a regular basis due to psychological states, and a tremendous amount of money is spent on the diagnosis and treatment of disorders that are manifestations of Mind Body Syndrome. If MBS were widely recognized by the lay public and medical professionals—both traditional and alternative practitioners—many people's symptoms could be alleviated, we would spend much less on health care, and we could prevent people from developing chronic symptom complexes that can cause tremendous suffering for decades.

The treatment of these disorders requires taking a careful history, judicious use of diagnostic tests to rule out serious pathological processes, attention to past and current psychosocial stressors and reactions to these stressors, validation of the real nature of the symptoms, explanation of the psychophysiological basis of the symptoms, and brief educational and psychological interventions. In these ways, patients are empowered to gain control over their symptoms, understand themselves better, and acquire tools to improve their physical and psychological health.

chapter 5

Do You Have Mind Body Syndrome?

It is more important to know what sort of person has the disease
than what kind of disease the person has. — Hippocrates

Tell me one last thing, said Harry. Is this real? Or has this been happening
inside my head?
Of course it is happening inside your head, Harry, but why on earth should
that mean that it is not real? — J.K. Rowling

How do you know if your pain or other symptoms are the result of Mind Body
Syndrome? First, you need to rule out tissue breakdown disorders that require biomedical treatments.
If you have had complete testing and no serious medical or physical disorder was found—no fractures,
no cancer, no heart disease, no infections, no nerve damage, no clear tissue pathology—then you
very likely have MBS.

Mind Body Syndrome does not cause cancer or heart disease or stroke. These are conditions
that increase in the population with increasing age and cause significant illness and, of course, often
death. These diseases are obviously tissue breakdown disorders, and there is no clear evidence that
they can be cured by changing how one thinks. As a physician, I recommend biomedical treatment
for people with these disorders. In addition, some people may also benefit from the techniques in
this book, i.e., techniques that are designed to calm the mind, which can cause physiological changes
in the body that can help with diabetes, heart disease and chronic lung diseases. And this program
can also help cope with common reactions to these disorders, such as anxiety or depression. Finally,
people with medical diseases can also develop MBS symptoms in response to the stress of having
those diseases. For example, people with heart disease or cancer can have pain, fatigue, or insomnia

due to MBS. Therefore, this program can help those symptoms as well.

There is another group of disorders that I do not consider to be a part of MBS. Representative disorders in this category include asthma, systemic lupus, rheumatoid arthritis, and multiple sclerosis. Although these disorders occur in younger people (as does MBS), these are also clearly tissue break-down disorders. It has been shown that stress and emotional reactions to stress can exacerbate these medical conditions. In fact, there is a well known area of medicine known as psychoneuroimmunology which has shown that changes in our stress levels and emotional states can cause real changes in the immune reactions in the body. This group of disorders are caused by alterations in immune functioning and there are some studies and many case reports demonstrating that the techniques in this program can be effective in reducing or even reversing the effects of these disorders. I also recommend continuing their medical treatments as long as necessary.

With those caveats, this program is primarily designed for those with MBS, those in whom there is no tissue breakdown process in the body, whose pain and other MBS symptoms are caused by learned neural circuits, stress, and fearful reactions to the symptoms. For such people, this program can offer the opportunity for a cure or a remission of symptoms.

Illustrative Stories

To prepare you for the kind of self-evaluation you will be doing, here are some cases I have encountered that illustrate some common patterns seen in the development of MBS:

A FORTY-FIVE-YEAR-OLD WOMAN *developed stomach pains and anxiety attacks in the fall one year after her husband died. He was terminally ill and, in accord with his wishes, she had to decide to disconnect his life support, which she felt was in conflict with her religious beliefs. Each fall, her pains returned and increased. Several GI specialists saw her, but no one could help her resolve her pain. Through this program, she learned that her feelings about her husband's death (primarily guilt and loss) caused her pain. Her anxiety attacks were generally in the afternoon, occuring almost exactly at the time of day that he died.*

A FIFTY-TWO-YEAR-OLD MAN *developed back pain while on a plane from Michigan to California, where he was living. As a child, his father was his hero and well liked by every-*

one in his small Michigan town. His mother was critical and self-absorbed. She demeaned the young boy constantly, and one day he replied to her in a disrespectful manner at home. Later that day, the mother called the local police and had him taken out of school in handcuffs and put into the town jail for the rest of the day, simply for talking back to his mother. After growing up, he moved to California. When he was fifty, he returned home to visit his father, who was now elderly and in a nursing home. Upon arriving home, he found that his mother was mistreating his father and he felt that his father was "imprisoned" in the nursing home. On the flight back, he developed severe back pains that lasted for 2 years.

A THIRTY-FOUR-YEAR-OLD MAN *was raised by a dominant father and a submissive mother in a small, very religious town. He was highly skilled in school and sports, and was admired by most people. When drunk, his father would often physically abuse his mother, but this was accepted as "normal" in his community and no action was ever taken. When asked how he felt about this, the patient replied that he often vowed that if he ever hit a woman, he would "cut off his hand." When he was a Ph.D. student, he was under the stress of preparing for his oral exams and was working feverishly on a big project. At this time, he began to have pain in both of his hands. The pain progressed to the point where he could not turn a doorknob, could not work on a computer, and could not pick up his infant son. Despite extensive testing and seeking care from several hand specialists, no one could explain his pain. When asked to recall any other events that occurred at the time of the onset of his pain, he noted that there was a conflict between two of his mentors. One mentor was a woman, who began to tell people that he was not fit to be in the Ph.D. program. He felt that she threatened his ability to complete his program. He was unaware of the depth of anger he felt towards her and his even stronger feelings of guilt at the prospect of his anger towards a woman. This internal and subconscious conflict was the trigger for his severe hand pain.*

A FORTY-TWO-YEAR-OLD WOMAN *grew up in a nurturing, close family within an idyllic rural community. Her mother chose to give her a larger share of the family inheritance, and this set off a contested will and the loss of her close relationships with her siblings. The trauma of those changes was enough to trigger severe back pain.*

The specific symptoms caused by MBS can be quite different, even though the stressor and the emotional reaction may be very similar to that which occurred in childhood, as shown by the following brief vignettes.

> A TEENAGER DEVELOPED HEADACHES *after being sexually abused by an older brother. She developed fibromyalgia later in life at a time when she was emotionally abused by her husband.*

> A WOMAN DEVELOPED MIGRAINE HEADACHES *as a child after her parents divorced and then developed interstitial cystitis as an adult after her own divorce.*

Sometimes MBS symptoms can be triggered by a positive event. In my own life, I developed neck pain after my daughter was born. She was our first child, and I was extremely happy at the time. However, her arrival complicated our lives. I was busy with work and busy at home, and my daughter didn't sleep well at night. I was up several times a night with her, walking up and down the stairs with her to get her back to sleep. After several months of this, my wife and I disagreed on how to deal with her crying at night. Now, in retrospect, I realize I felt stressed, resentful, and trapped. Not being able to express (or even recognize) these feelings, I developed neck pain, which persisted for several months.

Although many people with chronic pain, anxiety, or depression have histories of significant stressful life events, this is not always the case. I have seen countless people who have MBS who have had normal childhoods without significant trauma. I am one such person. MBS occurs in most people at least to some degree, especially those who are sensitive and tend to put pressure on themselves by being overly perfectionistic or having excessively high expectations for themselves. Individuals who put other's needs before their own and who have difficulty taking care of themselves or standing up for themselves are at particular risk for MBS.

It is important to understand that MBS is usually triggered by some kind of stressful situation and emotions related to that situation. But the situation may not be a major traumatic event; it may be a episode of sibling rivalry, a small social slight or a missed opportunity. It may be some events that don't even register or are not noted as significant. It just needs to be something just big enough to trigger the danger/alarm mechanism; and these kinds of events happen to most of us on a regular basis. Usually these symptoms resolve in a few minutes, hours or days. However, when we are paying close attention to such symptoms, the reaction of fear or worry can lead to further increase in activation of the danger/alarm mechanism.

This can easily create a cycle of pain-fear-pain, anxiety-fear-anxiety, or depression-fear-depression. And therefore, reversing the MBS symptoms doesn't always require identifying or processing the stressful life event or the emotions connected to it. It may be as simple as reprogramming the brain to reduce the danger/alarm mechanism and calm ourselves in the face of the MBS symptoms.

Common Mind Body Symptoms

We have found over the years that most of the people who have the chronic painful conditions and the other conditions that people seek out this program actually do have mind body or a condition caused by neural circuits in the brain. However, clearly not everyone does.

This section contains a list of some of the most common mind-body or neural circuit conditions. We will help you review your specific condition and situation in detail as part of this program. Most people will be able to recognize their situation as being a mind body or a neural circuit disorder easily. One of the most important components of this program is to help you understand what you have. In order to free yourself from chronic pain and these other associated conditions, it is necessary to know for certain that you do not have a structural condition, i.e., that your body is not broken or damaged. And that you can expect to recover by using this program

Before starting this program, everyone should have a complete and thorough medical evaluation to make sure that there is no structural condition that requires traditional medical attention. The following is a quick reference guide to some of the more common mind body or neural circuit conditions. There are two critical steps in making a diagnosis of one of these conditions: 1) ruling out a structural disorder and 2) ruling in MBS or a neural circuit condition. This list contains some information as a start in helping you achieve the first step, ruling out.

Tension and migraine headaches:

The medical causes of headaches include problems within the brain, such as brain tumors, brain aneurysms, and inflammation or infection in the brain (meningitis, encephalitis, vasculitis). There are also conditions that occur outside of the brain, such as sinus disorders, tooth disorders, and ear disorders. Once these serious medical disorders are ruled out by an examination, blood tests, and X-rays or MRIs, you can be assured that your headaches are due to a neural circuit condition. Tension headaches, cluster headaches, and occipital neuralgia are forms of MBS. Many people will tell you that your headaches are due to foods, weather, season, lights, sounds, or other external factors. However, these factors are not the cause of chronic headaches, they are events that trigger the danger mechanism to turn on headaches.

Irritable bowel syndrome (IBS) and chronic abdominal pain:

The diagnosis of IBS is only made when a structural condition, such as ulcerative colitis or Crohn's disease, has been ruled out. Therefore, IBS is not caused by any damage to the bowel. People with IBS have a variety of symptoms that are worsened by stress. This, of course, is the definition of a mind body condition. Please note that certain foods are not the cause of IBS or abdominal pain, unless you have been diagnosed with lactose intolerance or gluten enteropathy (celiac disease) based upon rigorous medical testing. We do not recommend eliminating foods in order to recover from IBS.

Neck and back pain:

Almost everyone has had some neck or back pain at some point in their life. It's common to get some degree of pain with overuse or with a sudden twist or pull. But these mild injuries will always heal and the pain will go away in a matter of a few hours or a day or two, at most. But when a very mild injury leads to pain that lingers for days or weeks, this is almost always MBS. The brain is continuing to create pain that was initially generated by the mild injury. Chronic neck or back pain can begin with an injury or can occur at any time randomly, such as waking up with pain. You didn't injure yourself during sleep! Your brain turned on pain due to some issues that were bothering you in your life, sometimes even if you're not aware of them.

We have stated that virtually all MRIs are abnormal. Very few people have an MRI of their back or neck that is perfectly normal. Even teenagers and those in their 20s and 30s usually have some abnormalities on a neck or back MRI. And here, we are talking about all people, i.e., people with no pain at all! Bulging discs and degenerating discs are actually normal findings and are not the cause of pain. Even people with herniated discs often have no pain. The same is true for spinal stenosis and slipped vertebrae (spondylolisthesis). Many doctors will likely tell you that these common findings are the cause of your neck or back pain. That is not necessarily true and we will show you how to figure that out.

If your MRI shows a fracture, an infection, evidence of an inflammatory condition such as ankylosing spondylitis, or a tumor, then medical treatment is necessary. If there is a huge herniated disc that causes pain, numbness in the specific area of your arm or leg associated with that nerve, and there is muscle weakness (such as a foot drop) or loss of the associated reflex in the leg, then that disc could be the problem. But surgery is rarely necessary even in that situation, as the vast majority of those very large disc problems will heal on their own.

Having surgery for chronic low back pain in the absence of the large disc problem mentioned above is not a good idea. That kind of surgery is very invasive, it often doesn't help, it can lead to complications, and it can even make the pain worse. Be very careful if a back surgeon tells you that they can fix your chronic low back pain or chronic neck pain (in the absence of pain in the arm or leg)!

Fibromyalgia:

The name, fibromyalgia, means that there is pain that is widespread and chronic. It does not imply that there is a specific structural problem. In fact, the diagnosis of fibromyalgia can only be made when structural conditions are ruled out. A doctor will typically do tests to rule out rheumatoid arthritis or lupus. In summary, fibromyalgia is a mind body condition, even though there are many theories linking it to physical causes. None of those supposed causes have been validated to date.

Osteoarthritis:

Osteoarthritis (OA) is the term used for the "wear and tear" arthritis that occurs with increasing age. Everyone has some X-ray evidence of OA with age. But these X-ray findings usually occur without causing pain. Be wary of doctors who tell you that your knee, shoulder or hip pain is caused by OA, just because the X-ray shows OA. Even X-rays that show "bone on bone" arthritis can be misleading and not be the cause of pain. Of course, some people will get severe OA of their joints and may require joint replacements. Before concluding that OA is the problem make sure to investigate the pain. This program will give you information on how to do this kind of investigation of pain (as we mentioned above, step two, or ruling in MBS). For example, if the joint pain comes and goes, is much better on some days, is triggered by weather or stress, these are all signs of mind-body pain, rather than OA pain.

Pelvic pain syndromes:

There are a wide range of conditions that are often diagnosed when someone has chronic pelvic pain. Depending on the location and type of the pain, these are some of the terms used to describe the pain: pudendal neuralgia, pelvic floor dysfunction, vulvodynia, coccydynia, interstitial cystitis, chronic prostatitis and others. Just like the situation with fibromyalgia, these terms only describe the

the pain: pudendal neuralgia, pelvic floor dysfunction, vulvodynia, coccydynia, interstitial cystitis, chronic prostatitis and others. Just like the situation with fibromyalgia, these terms only describe the problem, in essence, saying: "You have pain." But none of these terms actually imply any structural damage at all. When any of these diagnoses are made, it means that this is a mind body condition. As with all other conditions, you can prove that it's a mind body condition by doing the investigation which we will describe.

Endometriosis is a condition where there is tissue from the lining of the uterus located outside of the uterus, usually in the pelvic region, around the fallopian tubes or ovaries. Doctors will look for this condition as part of an evaluation for pelvic pain. However, many doctors will not tell you that many women have evidence of endometriosis without having pain at all. Just as in the situation with OA, endometriosis is often not the actual cause of the pain. You can figure this out by a careful investigation of the symptoms as will be described.

Heartburn/GERD (gastro-esophageal reflux disorder):

This is a very common condition that can occur due to stomach material going up into the esophagus or throat. Everyone has had this occur at times. It leaves a sour taste in the mouth or causes some mild burning behind the sternum (breastbone). It is a transient condition almost all of the time. In a few people, it can be more severe and cause more frequent symptoms. However, the brain can generate all of these sensations in the absence of any actual material escaping from the stomach. These symptoms can be easily assessed by standard testing, including an EGD or barium swallow. Sometimes a pH monitor can be placed as well. If these tests are normal, then you do not have GERD. The vast majority of people with actual heartburn can be helped by using an acid blocking medication. If these medications are not working, then the problem is not GERD: It is more likely to be a mind body condition. Even when those medications work, they might be working due to the placebo effect. So, use the investigation methods we will describe below to be certain of the correct diagnosis.

Tinnitus:

Ringing in the ears (tinnitus) will occur after going to a very loud rock concert or being exposed to very loud sounds for several hours. This is a normal reaction and will go away in a day or so. Tinnitus can also occur in the absence of any ear damage due to a mind-body condition. Usually, this occurs when there is something upsetting going on in one's life, but it can occur for a few minutes on a random basis. Persistent ringing in the ear is almost always due to a neural circuit or mind body condition, unless there is definite damage causing hearing loss and imbalance.

Dizziness and vertigo:

Lightheadedness and the sensation of the room spinning (vertigo) are common conditions that occur on occasion in many people. If they are persistent, they are usually due to a mind body condition. Medical testing can rule out any problem with the brain, heart or ears.

POTS (postural orthostatic tachycardia syndrome):

This is a condition in which people have dizziness when they stand up and a rapid heartbeat. It was initially thought to be due to some kind of heart condition but further investigation has shown this to be a mind body condition.

Muscle tics and spasms:

These are common conditions that are almost always due to the brains' neural circuits, rather than any disease. The muscles or nerves are not damaged, they are being activated by the brain. Dystonias also fall into this category.

Non-epileptic seizures (PNEA—paroxysmal non-epileptic attacks):

This is a condition in which the person looks like they are having a seizure, but in reality they are not. It is always a mind-body condition. This is easily diagnosed by doing an EEG/video monitor test in a neurology unit.

Acute loss of voice (aphasia) or change in voice pattern (spasmodic dysphonia):

These are almost always neural circuit conditions. Medical testing will rule out any specific vocal cord or neurologic disorder.

Brain fog and inattention syndromes:

It is common for the brain to create these conditions. A specific neurologic disorder such as ADHD or dementia needs to be ruled out. Most people have lapses of memory that are not worrisome and should not be taken to imply that they are "losing their mind." Even significant inability to concentrate and remember things are usually due to a mind body condition.

Tingling and numbness sensations:

It is common to have unusual sensations on the skin. These often occur in the hands or feet, but can occur anywhere in the body. Itching is another common condition. Medical testing, as always, is necessary to rule out actual nerve damage due to vitamin deficiencies, chemotherapy or an alcohol use disorder. When a diagnosis of small fiber neuropathy is made, you can be assured that it is a mind body condition, as the nerves are actually working well. Many people are also told that they have idiopathic neuropathy. If there is no evidence of nerve damage based upon the neurologic exam, you can be assured that this is a neural circuit condition. EMG testing often shows some mild "damage," but just like MRIs, these findings are usually seen in normal people without pain. Even skin biopsies said to be diagnostic of small fiber neuropathy are seen in normal people.

TMJ (temporo-mandibular joint) disorder:

TMJ disorder is a common condition that is presumed to be due to teeth clenching/grinding and/or damage to the joint when the jaw meets the skull. However, research shows that people with teeth clenching and grinding at night do not have TMJ pain any more than other people do. The findings of damage to the TM joint are also seen in people who have no pain. This is usually a mind body condition, when it is investigated carefully.

Urinary frequency/Interstitial cystitis (IC):

Frequent urination and bladder pains are common conditions that are rarely due to structural damage. Studies show that there is often evidence of mild bladder damage in normal people who have cystoscopies. Diets to avoid certain foods usually lead to more problems than solutions, and are not necessary.

Palpitations:

Many people have palpitations of the heart due to skipped beats or extra beats. These are almost always benign conditions that can be due to stress. Cardiac testing should be done to rule out any more serious conditions such as atrial fibrillation or ventricular tachycardia, which require medical treatment.

Facial pain/trigeminal neuralgia:

This condition is almost always due to neural circuits rather than any structural damage. Testing may show some compression of the facial nerve by arteries or veins, but this finding is common in those who have no pain. Careful investigation is helpful to prove a mind body cause.

Complex regional pain syndrome (CRPS):

This condition used to be called RSD, or reflex sympathetic dystrophy. It consists of pain and some-times skin changes in a hand or foot. It may involve an arm or leg as well. Even though it can seem to be a structural problem due to the color changes (red or purple) or the skin changes (heat, cold or swelling), it has been shown to be reversible using a mind body approach.

Eating disorders:

Anorexia, bulimia, and overeating disorders are common and almost never found to be due to some underlying brain or medical condition. They are also mind body disorders.

Anxiety/Obsessive-compulsive disorder (OCD):

The various types of anxiety disorders, including generalized anxiety, social anxiety, phobias and OCD, are almost always due to a mind-body condition. Excess thyroid hormone (hyperthyroidism) should be ruled out.

Depression:

Depression is also almost always a mind-body condition. Hypothyroidism, very low testosterone levels (in men) and a few other hormonal conditions should be ruled out. Menopause is not a cause of depression from a hormonal standpoint.

There is some controversy about anxiety, OCD, and depression. Most doctors currently believe that these are conditions in which there are some kind of abnormalities in the brain, basically, some kind of brain damage. Therefore, people who suffer from these disorders are being told that they need medications to recover and that they will often need those medications for their whole life. They have been told that they have a problem with some of the neurotransmitters, such as serotonin, or that they have inflammation or a genetic condition. None of these explanations have been proven to be correct. The truth is that these conditions are mind body or neural circuit disorders that are reversible by using the methods in this program.

Post-COVID syndrome/long haul COVID:

About 10% of people who have had COVID-19 have developed a variety of symptoms, such as short-ness of breath, fatigue, headache, brain fog and others. Many of the people with this condition have never even had COVID-19 or had only mild cases. There has been a tremendous amount of stress and fear during these last few years and it is highly likely that most of the people suffering with this condition have no structural disorder and can be helped by a mind body approach.

There are many, many more syndromes that are commonly diagnosed as mind body disorders. For a complete list, see the book on the diagnosis of common mind body conditions published by the Psychophysiologic Disorders Association, PPDAssociation.org.

Mind Body Syndrome Self-Diagnosis

To figure out if you have MBS and what issues in your life may have contributed to this disorder, take the time to complete the work sheets below. They will help you understand yourself better, and this understanding is the key to ridding yourself of your pain. This section is based upon the detailed interview I use with my patients.

STEP 1: RULING OUT A MEDICAL CONDITION

The following list of symptoms and diagnoses are likely to be caused by MBS (though some of them can also be caused by other medical conditions that can be easily ruled out by your physician). The more of these you have had during your lifetime, the more likely it is that you have MBS. People with several of these conditions have usually seen many doctors and been given multiple diagnoses, but their doctors have not considered MBS. This is because biotechnological medical practice tends to look at each body system in isolation. You may have seen a neurologist, orthopedic surgeon or neurosurgeon, gastroenterologist, rheumatologist, or others. But no one is looking at the whole person. MBS occurs in people, not in body parts, and we can only understand it by evaluating the whole person, the mind, and the body.

Ruling out a structural condition is usually relatively straight-forward. Many conditions are clearly MBS, such as irritable bowel syndrome, non-ulcer dyspepsia, migraine and tension headaches, CRPS (complex regional pain syndrome), fibromyalgia, POTS (postural orthostatic tachycardia syndrome), myofascial pain syndrome, multiple chemical sensitivities and irritable bladder syndrome (interstitial cystitis). Many other conditions are usually MBS and simple testing can rule out a serious problem, such as the case with chronic tendonitis, numbness, burning and tingling sensations, chest pains, palpitations, pelvic pain syndromes, insomnia, chronic abdominal pain, tinnitus, dizziness, repetitive strain injury, anxiety, depression, and chronic fatigue syndrome. For the majority of people with chronic neck and back pain, the correct diagnosis is MBS, although few doctors, physical therapists and chiropractors will be aware of this. As long as the X-rays and MRIs do not show a tumor, infection, inflammatory condition, or fracture, and if the neurological examination is normal to rule out nerve damage, the presence of degenerative discs, spurs, facet problems, and bulging discs should not be interpreted to be causing pain.

CHECK EACH ITEM ON THE FOLLOWING LIST and write down at what age you were when each set of symptoms first appeared in your life.

Date of onset:

1. Heartburn, acid reflux _____

2. Abdominal pains _____

3. Irritable bowel syndrome _____

4. Tension headaches _____

5. Migraine headaches _____

6. Unexplained rashes _____

7. Anxiety and/or panic attacks

_____

8. Depression _____

9. Obsessive-compulsive thought patterns

_____

10. Eating disorders _____

11. Insomnia or trouble sleeping _____

12. Fibromyalgia _____

13. Back pain _____

14. Neck pain _____

15. Shoulder pain _____

16. Repetitive strain injury _____

17. Carpal tunnel syndrome _____

18. Complex regional pain syndrome (CRPS)

_____

Date of onset:

19. Temporomandibular joint syndrome

    (TMJ) _____

20. Chronic tendonitis _____

21. Facial pain _____

22. Numbness, tingling sensations _____

23. Fatigue or chronic fatigue syndrome

    _____

24. Palpitations _____

25. Chest pain _____

26. Hyperventilation _____

27. Interstitial cystitis/spastic bladder (irritable

    bladder syndrome) _____

28. Pelvic pain _____

29. Muscle tenderness _____

30. Postural orthostatic tachycardia syndrome

    (POTS) _____

31. Tinnitus _____

32. Dizziness _____

33. PTSD _____

34. Multiple chemical sensitivities

    _____

There are many reasons why many people and their doctors ignore or reject the whole idea of a mind body connection. Here are two myths about chronic pain for you to understand.

MYTH #1: AN OLD INJURY CAN BE THE CAUSE OF PAIN

It is so common for people to think that an injury that occurred weeks, months or even years ago is the reason that they have pain now. This idea is not true. All injuries heal. We know that. We have not existed as people on this earth for hundreds of thousands of years to have pain after an injury heals. We would never have survived. Every cut or bruise you have had has healed. Our bodies do this; every single time. An injury can clearly cause pain, but pain that persists after an injury heals is not due to lack of healing, it is due to the brain continuing to create that pain; nothing more. These are neural circuits; not lack of healing.

Sometimes doctors will tell you that an old injury is the source of your pain because there is a misalignment or that the tissues are inflamed or that there is a scar there. These are not actually true. Everyone has some misalignments in their body, such as a leg that is longer, a curve of the spine, or a hip or shoulder that is higher than the other one. But we are made to adjust to these and to not get pain from them. Doctors often tell people that their posture is bad and that is the source of their pain. This is not true either. Posture doesn't matter that much and this has been shown in many research studies.

Scars do not cause pain. There are no nerve fibers in scars to cause pain. Therefore, pain that is in the area of a scar is MBS. Scars can heal in ways that cause some disfigurement, such as burn scars on the skin that can cause fingers to be contracted, but while this may limit mobility, it is not the cause of pain. Internal scarring can occasionally cause some degree of obstruction of the bowel, which can be painful when it occurs, but this is rarely the cause of ongoing pain.

MYTH #2: PAIN IS CAUSED BY INFLAMMATION THAT CANNOT BE SEEN

There are two kinds of inflammation: macro-inflammation that you can see and micro-inflammation that cannot be seen. Macro-inflammation occurs with a strep throat or an infected cut or gout or rheumatoid arthritis. You can see the redness, swelling, heat and sometimes pus. This is tissue damage that usually causes pain.

However, some doctors tell people that their pain is due to inflammation that they cannot see, such as in the tissues or joints or muscles. These areas may even be tender to touch. But, do not be fooled. Everyone has micro-inflammation in their body to some degree. Tests for this kind of inflammation, such as an ESR or CRP, can be elevated in many people, especially people who have pain or a lot of stress in their lives. But this type of inflammation is not the cause of pain.

STEP 2: RULING IN A MIND BODY CONDITION

Once a structural condition is ruled out, one should look carefully at the symptoms to **rule in** a mind body disorder. This can be accomplished by understanding the characteristics of neural circuits. Neural circuits are learned by the brain and usually have specific characteristics that give us clues to the true nature of the symptoms. For example, pain that goes away when one is on vacation and returns when getting home fits much better with MBS than a medical condition. There are a set of these types of clues that we use to confirm the diagnosis of a mind body condition. Essentially, we are able to rule in MBS when these clues are present. We can group these clues into three categories: Functional, Inconsistent and Triggered, which I call the FIT criteria.

There are many reasons why many people and their doctors ignore or reject the whole idea of a mind body connection. Here are two myths about chronic pain for you to understand:

Functional: This means that the symptoms of MBS do not fit with and are not explainable by known structural conditions.

Symptoms begin without a physical precipitation (often occurring with no injury, upon waking up in the morning, or during a time of stress)

Symptoms persist after an injury has healed (all injuries heal and scars do not cause pain)

Symptoms are in a distribution pattern that is symmetric in the body, mirror image on the left and right side (this rarely occurs with structural pain)

Symptoms occur on one whole side of the body or occur on half of the face, head, or torso (this does not fit into a pattern that corresponds to physical damage)

Symptoms spread over time to different areas of the body

Symptoms radiate to the opposite side of the body or down a whole leg or arm (unlike a nerve pain that would only affect the part of the arm or leg where that nerve is located)

Symptoms that occur in many different body parts at the same time

Symptoms that have the quality of tingling, electric, burning, numb, hot or cold (these are commonly MBS, especially when there is no evidence for actual nerve damage)

Inconsistent: This means that the symptoms vary in ways that a structural condition would not.

Symptoms shift from one location in the body to another, either within hours, days or weeks at a time

Symptoms are more or less intense depending on the time of day, or occur first thing in the morning or in the middle of the night (this is due to subconscious brain activity)

Symptoms occur after, but not during, activity or exercise (a structural injury hurts when used and is better when rested)

Symptoms occur when one thinks about them or when someone asks about it

Symptoms occur when stress is increased or one thinks about stressful situations

Symptoms are minimal or non-existent when engaged in joyful or distracting activities, such as when on vacation or when not thinking about the symptoms

Symptoms are minimal or non-existent after some kind of therapy, such as massage, chiropractic, Reiki, acupuncture, an herbal or vitamin supplement (anything that calms the danger signal will tend to decrease symptoms)

Triggered: This means that the symptoms are brought on by stimuli that would not actually cause the symptom physically, but they activate the brain to generate the symptom.

Symptoms are triggered by things that are not related to the actual symptom, such as foods, smells, sounds, light, computer screens, menses, changes in the weather (weather has been shown in research to not increase pain, despite what most people think) or specific movements

Symptoms are triggered by the anticipation of stress, such as prior to school, work, a doctor's visit, a medical test, a visit to a relative, or a social gathering; or during those activities

Symptoms that are triggered by simply **imagining** engaging in the triggering activity, such as bending over, turning the neck, sitting or standing (this is a great exercise to diagnose MBS as it confirms that the brain is creating pain in the absence of actually performing the activity)

Symptoms are triggered by light touch or innocuous stimuli, such as the wind or cold (people with MBS are often overly sensitive to touch. Light touch doesn't actually affect the deeper body part where the pain is being felt)

Most people with MBS have several of these features that make it easy to rule this condition in. Even if only one of the above characteristics is present, that will be enough to confirm the diagnosis of MBS. It only takes one clear piece of evidence for a detective, such as Sherlock Holmes, to crack the case. The same is true for the diagnosis of MBS.

There are several other common features of MBS. Most people with MBS have had a significant amount of stressful life events, especially in childhood, but this is variable. I did not have an unhappy childhood, yet I have had many episodes of MBS over the years. They often have many different types of MBS symptoms over the years. When someone has had many of these, it is very likely that their current issues are also MBS (assuming that there is no clear and specific structural disorder), although some people just have one MBS symptom. The onset of MBS usually occurs in connection with a significant life stressor, although sometimes this is not the case, or the stressor seems relatively small. And they usually have many of the personality traits associated with MBS. In this next section, you will be completing an assessment of your situation to help you discover why you have MBS.

STEP 3: INVESTIGATE YOUR CHILDHOOD

Now consider the following questions and write brief answers to as many of them as seem important.

What words would you use to describe your father?

(Substitute another caregiver if you didn't grow up with your father.)

_____

_____

What kind of work did your father do? Was he successful in his career?

_____

Was your father loving? Did he hug you or tell you he loved you? Was he supportive?

_____

Were you particularly close to your father? Did he confide in you?

_____

Was his love conditional?

_____

Did your father have high expectations of you?

_____

Was he critical or judgmental?

_____

Was he a perfectionist?

_____

Did he yell at you?

_____

Did he hit or punish you?

_____

Were you afraid of him?

_____

Was your father aloof, neglectful, or self-centered?

_____

Were some children given preferential treatment or treated more harshly than others?
If so, how did that make you feel? How did that affect the relationship between you and any of
your siblings?

_____

_____

Did your father drink or use drugs? If so, how did that affect him, the family, and you?

_____

Did your father have any mental health issues?

_____

Was he anxious, worried, or insecure?

_____

How did your father treat your mother?

_____

Did you identify with your father?

_____

Did you attempt to be like him or to be different from him?

_____

What words would you use to describe your mother (or another caregiver)?

_____

_____

What kind of work did your mother do?

_____

Was she successful in her career?

_____

Was your mother loving? Did she hug you or tell you she loved you? Was she supportive?

_____

_____

Were you particularly close to your mother? Did she confide in you?

_____

Was her love conditional?

_____

Did your mother have high expectations of you?

_____

Was she critical or judgmental?

_____

Was she a perfectionist?

_____

Did she yell at you?

_____

Did she hit or punish you?

_____

Were you afraid of her?

_____

Was your mother aloof, neglectful, or self-centered?

_____

Were some children given preferential treatment or treated more harshly than others? If so, how did that make you feel? How did that affect the relationship between you and any of your siblings?

_____

Was she anxious, worried, or insecure?

_____

Did you identify with your mother?

_____

Did you attempt to be like her or to be different from her?

_____

How did your mother treat your father?

_____

Who was in charge of the house?

_____

Who handled disciplinary issues?

_____

Did your parents argue?

_____

Did anyone other than your mother and father have responsibility for you or care for you as a child?
If so, who?

_____

Repeat the above questions for these individuals if they had significant roles in your upbringing.
Use separate paper for these questions.

Think of the relationships you had with your siblings while you were growing up.
Were there resentments or jealousies?

_____

_____

Was there any cruelty, meanness, or abuse?

_____

Did any of your siblings have any illnesses, psychological problems, or drug abuse problems?

_____

Did any of your siblings rebel, act out, or behave in ways that were upsetting to your parents or to you?

_____

How did you react to these situations?

_____

How was money handled in your family?

_____

Did you feel that money was a scarce resource?

_____

Did your parents use money as a controlling agent?

_____

Were they generous with money or not?

_____

Did you work as a child or teenager?

_____

Finally, consider if there were any particularly stressful or traumatic events in your childhood.
Describe any of the following: deaths, moves, bullying, taunting, teasing, emotional or physical abuse, changes in school situations, conflicts with teachers, or changes in family situations?

_____
_____
_____
_____
_____
_____
_____
_____

Have you ever been subjected to any episodes of unwanted sexual activity or sexual abuse?

_____
_____
_____

Childhood experiences create very powerful reactions in our minds that remain for the rest of our lives. Emotions that are generated when we are young can very easily get triggered later in life, and, when they are triggered, can cause the start of Mind Body Syndrome. It is usually relatively easy to identify the childhood issues that people with MBS have grown up with.

It is well known that a large percentage of the people with irritable bowel syndrome, fibromyalgia, TMJ syndrome, and other MBS illnesses have been neglected or abused—sexually, emotionally, or physically—as children or adolescents. People who have suffered from severe childhood abuse are most likely to have many forms of MBS.

I saw a woman whose mother was a prostitute and a cocaine addict and whose father was a heroin addict who sexually abused and even tortured her. She became a prostitute and a cocaine addict as an adolescent. She eventually went to jail, broke her addiction to drugs, and was able to raise a daughter and find a job. However, over all those years of traumatic experiences, she developed fibromyalgia, migraine headaches, irritable bowel syndrome, TMJ syndrome, chronic fatigue, back pain, insomnia, anxiety, depression, and several other MBS disorders.

Not everyone with MBS has had severe childhood traumas, however. For many people, the childhood issues that generate strong emotions are normal childhood experiences. How many of us have felt jealous of a sibling or ostracized by friends in middle school or picked on by a bully in elementary school? These common experiences can also generate enough emotions to cause MBS syndrome, either at the time of the events or, more commonly, later in life.

I treated a woman who grew up with loving parents but with a difficult younger sister. Her sister was constantly in trouble, and my patient was always covering up for her, even though she resented her sister lying and avoiding responsibilities. When my patient was thirty-three years old, she was leading a team at work in an important project. One woman on the team avoided her share of the work and tried to cover up her lack of effort. My patient was trapped in a situation eerily similar to that of dealing with her younger sister and had to double her work to get the project completed. During that time, she developed back pain because the situation at work triggered the stored emotional reactions from her youth. Several years later, she developed headaches every time she drove across town to visit her father, who was in a nursing home that her sister had selected for its proximity to her. After learning of her life story, it became clear that her resentment of her sister was the underlying trigger for the back pain and headaches.

STEP 4: CORE ISSUES

Once you have carefully and honestly reviewed the stresses in your life, you will likely begin to see patterns. You will be able to identify your "core issues," those issues that have been stored in your subconscious mind and that are most likely to trigger the onset of physical and psychological symptoms. Indicate which of the following patterns apply to you, or describe any other patterns that apply to you.

1. Loss and abandonment (losing a parent or sibling, divorce, moving) _____

2. Childhood abuse or neglect (physical, sexual, emotional abuse; never feeling loved or cared for) _____

3. Not fitting in or feeling ostracized (being teased or picked on, being shy and reserved, not being athletic or popular) _____

4. Feeling pressure to succeed or be perfect (from parents, other family members, church or religious organizations, or self) _____

5. Feeling inferior to siblings or other relatives (not as beautiful, funny, athletic, interesting, accomplished) _____

6. Never feeling good enough, having to "earn" love from parents, feeling criticized much of the time _____

7. Resentment and/or anger towards family members, religious leaders, neighbors _____

8. Learning to be anxious, worried, or insecure _____

9. Identifying with one or several family members and trying to emulate them; trying to be different from one or several family members _____

10. Learning that others were more important than you; that you should never put yourself first, never stand up for yourself or express your true feelings _____

11. Other patterns _____

_____

_____

_____

STEP 5: PERSONALITY TRAITS

These factors are commonly seen in people with MBS. Check those that apply to you. Would you describe yourself as:

1. Having low self-esteem _____

2. Being a perfectionist _____

3. Having high expectations of yourself _____

4. Wanting to be good and/or be liked _____

5. Frequently feeling guilt _____

6. Feeling dependent on others _____

7. Being conscientious _____

8. Being hard on yourself _____

9. Being overly responsible _____

10. Having difficulty making decisions _____

11. Following rules strictly _____

12. Having difficulty letting go _____

13. Feeling cautious, shy, or reserved _____

14. Tending to hold thoughts and feelings in _____

15. Tending to harbor rage or resentment _____

16. Not standing up for yourself or express your true feelings _____

Conflict in one's mind is a very important part of the mechanism that creates and perpetuates MBS. The traits above are aspects of the conscience—they are things that we feel obligated to do or ways we feel obligated to be. Most people with MBS are people who try hard, who care what others think of them, who want to be good and want to be liked. They tend to be conscientious, responsible, and hard on themselves. These personality traits are generally found in good people, people you would like to know and be friends with. The problem is that people like this put extra pressure on themselves. They tend to get down on themselves and beat themselves up for their failings. When external events and stressors occur and we compound the stress by putting more pressure on ourselves, we are much more likely to develop MBS.

STEP 6: FINDING CONNECTIONS BETWEEN LIFE STRESSES, CORE ISSUES, AND THE ONSET OF MBS SYMPTOMS

Once you have identified your core issues, review the list of potential MBS symptoms in Step 1, on page 73. On the next page, list the times in your life when you developed any of the MBS manifestations in chronological order. Think carefully about what events occurred just prior to or during the onset of symptoms. You will typically find that the symptoms began at or shortly after you experienced something that was stressful and that reminded you of your core issues (triggering your emotional speed dial), and you felt trapped in that situation. List each symptom, then write down the triggering events or situations, and the emotions and/or core issues which caused the symptoms to occur.

Age	MBS symptom(s) (from Step 1)	Potential triggering events	Emotions that were triggered/core issues
___	_____	_____	_____
___	_____	_____	_____
___	_____	_____	_____
___	_____	_____	_____
___	_____	_____	_____
___	_____	_____	_____
___	_____	_____	_____
___	_____	_____	_____
___	_____	_____	_____
___	_____	_____	_____
___	_____	_____	_____
___	_____	_____	_____
___	_____	_____	_____
___	_____	_____	_____
___	_____	_____	_____
___	_____	_____	_____
___	_____	_____	_____
___	_____	_____	_____
___	_____	_____	_____
___	_____	_____	_____
___	_____	_____	_____
___	_____	_____	_____
___	_____	_____	_____
___	_____	_____	_____
___	_____	_____	_____
___	_____	_____	_____
___	_____	_____	_____
___	_____	_____	_____

When you place the symptoms and diagnoses that have occurred next to the life stressors, see what patterns emerge and what connections you can make. This is a critical step in figuring out why you have MBS. Do this for each of your MBS symptoms. For each symptom, think carefully about what was going on in your life at the time this symptom began. What events had occurred that bothered you? What emotions did you feel? How were these events or emotions similar to those you experienced in childhood? Which core issues might have been triggered? Did you feel trapped in some way, either physically or verbally?

Be as open and honest as you can in this process. Often it is very obvious that stressful life events in childhood have created the emotional memories of hurt, loss, fear, guilt, or anger, and it is equally obvious that certain stressors later in life triggered MBS symptoms.

However, sometimes it takes a fair amount of introspection and searching to find the connections. It is common for mild stressors in adult life to trigger significant symptoms if the stressor is related to earlier stressors, particularly from childhood. Neglect or lack of love by a parent can create a childhood hurt that can get triggered later in life by seemingly mild interactions. This pattern occurs because emotional memory is permanent and early childhood hurts create a reservoir of emotional pain. During the course of our lives, this emotional pain may build over time when new emotional hurts occur, especially those that are similar in nature to the earlier ones. Later in life, our bodies can easily react to a seemingly small emotional stressor, such as not getting a particular position, conflict with a colleague or boss, having a child or getting married, since that current stressor is linked in our subconscious mind to all of the earlier emotional issues. This process explains why a large emotional hurt in childhood may not produce any symptoms while a small stressor later in life can produce severe MBS.

While completing the table on the previous page, consider the following list for the primary emotions that were triggered: anger and resentment, fear, guilt, shame, sadness and loss.

Making Your Decision

For many people, doing these exercises will make it clear to you that you do have MBS. If you have been able to **rule out** a clearly identified structural disorder and then **ruled in** a neural circuit condition by using the FIT criteria in Step 1, you can be certain that you do have MBS. The exercises in the following steps can help you to understand why you have MBS, but they are not necessary for making the diagnosis. As I have stated, many people can have MBS without having obvious stressful situations or trauma in their life.

One young woman I evaluated had experienced severe childhood traumas and consequently had developed a very long list of disorders, including iritable bowel syndrome, anxiety, depression, neck pain, TMJ disorder, and fibromyalgia. She had been treated unsuccessfully for many years and was convinced that she was in a hopeless situation. After reviewing the clear connections between her life events and the onset of her MBS symptoms, she suddenly looked up at me and said, "I have Mind Body Syndrome." The certainty and confidence in her voice were striking, as she realized at that moment that she could take control of her life and shed these disorders that seemed incurable.

However, if you're not sure if you have MBS, or that your life experiences are actually the cause of your pain, consider these steps:

• Make sure you have seen a doctor and that you have had enough testing to rule out a purely physical cause for your pain and/or other symptoms.

• Discuss these issues with a counselor, relative, or good friend to help uncover the connections between the stresses in your life and your symptoms.

• Do further reading. I recommend reading one of Dr. John Sarno's landmark books, such as the *The Mindbody Prescription* or *The Divided Mind*. Dr. Sarno is a pioneer in this field, and this book describes how the MBS syndrome works (his term for it is Tension Myositis Syndrome). There are a number of other useful books listed in the appendix, such as David Clarke's *They Can't Find Anything Wrong*, Nancy Selfridge's *Freedom From Fibromyalgia*, David Hanscom's *Back in Control*, David Schechter's *Think Away Your Pain*, and Georgina Oldfield's, *Chronic Pain: Your Key to Recovery*.

• See a doctor or psychologist who specializes in MBS. The PPD/TMS Peer Network (tmswiki.org) is an excellent patient-run website with up-to-date information on MBS. The Psychophysiologic Disorders Association (PPDA, PPDAssociation.org) is a non-profit organization of medical professionals who have a commitment to bringing scientifically valid information about the mind body connection to the public and health care providers. There are excellent resources on both of these websites, including lists of practitioners who are well-versed in neural circuit disorders. In addition, the Pain Reprocessing Therapy

Institute has a list of practitioners who can diagnose and treat MBS, see painreprocessingtherapy.com. My website, unlearnyourpain.com, has a great deal of information in written and video formats. Click on the Media tab at the top of unlearnyourpain.com and link to any of the articles, lectures, podcasts and videos. In particular, there are a set of six animated videos that provide an explanation of neural circuit disorders that you can show to friends or family members to help them better understand this work. If you would like to make an appointment with me, you can contact me on my website: www.unlearnyourpain.com.

Creating Your Evidence Sheet

It has taken a lot of hard work to go through this process, but it will be worth it. You are taking a very important step towards recovery: knowing what the problem is. As you proceed through the program, you will refer back to this step over and over. You will review the facts that demonstrate that you have MBS, and nothing else. Since understanding that you have MBS is often counterintuitive and is at odds with traditional medical diagnoses, it can be useful to compile the evidence that confirms the diagnosis of MBS in one place.

A simple way to do this is to create an evidence sheet. Use the following lines to put together all of the evidence from the worksheets in this chapter that confirm MBS. Keep this list and refer back to it when you begin to doubt that you have MBS. Doubt about having MBS is common as our brain often falls back into fear and worry as we will see. Referring back to this list will help you quell those doubts, which will help you succeed in this program.

List of symptoms and syndromes that are typical of MBS: (on page 73)

_____

List of normal tests and evaluations that have ruled out a structural cause:

_____

List of items from the Functional criteria that confirm MBS: (on page 75)

_____

List of items from the Inconsistent criteria that confirm MBS: (on page 76)

_____

List of items from the Triggered criteria that confirm MBS: (on page 76)

_____

List of items from the personality traits criteria that suggest MBS: (on pages 83 and 84)

_____

List of items from the worksheet on connections between life stresses, core issues, and onset of MBS symptoms that confirm MBS: (on page 85)

_____

Once you have the correct diagnosis and you can say to yourself, "I have Mind Body Syndrome," you are ready to use the rest of this book to heal yourself. If you participate in this program, it is very likely that you will reduce or eliminate your MBS symptoms, increase your understanding of yourself, and learn how to gain control and mastery over your mind and body. In fact, the program has been so helpful that many people who have taken the program recommend it to everyone they know, including those who do not have symptoms of MBS.

chapter 6

Starting the Program:
The Power is in Your Hands

You never find yourself until you face the truth. — Pearl Bailey

To be nobody—but yourself—in a world which is doing its best, night and day, to make you everybody else—means to fight the hardest battle which any human being can fight; and never stop fighting. — e. e. cummings

The remainder of this book consists of a guide to curing yourself of Mind Body Syndrome. It is based upon the live, in-person program that I teach to individuals with MBS and is therefore designed to be completed in four weeks. However, one advantage of completing the program in book form is that you can do the exercises at your own pace.

This program is designed for those who have MBS. As mentioned before, it is not designed for those with pain or other symptoms caused by cancer, fractures, infections, or inflammatory diseases. Symptoms caused by MBS can be cured by doing this program. The most important factors in getting better are the belief that you do, in fact, have Mind Body Syndrome, understanding what factors in your life have caused the stresses and emotions that have triggered the symptoms of MBS (although that is not always obvious or even necessary), and learning how to reverse the neural circuits of pain, fatigue, anxiety and depression. It is my experience that those who do not have this belief and these understandings have a much more difficult time in ridding themselves of MBS. If you have significant doubts about whether your symptoms are caused by MBS, consider the advice given at the end of chapter 5. However, many people are unsure if they have MBS or if it explains all of their symptoms. You may doubt if this program will work for you. You may not have a clear sense of what events in your life caused your symptoms. I often see people in this predicament. My suggestion is to go ahead and begin the program. Over time, you will likely see that the symptoms vary in ways that inform you that they are, in fact, due to MBS. The methods I describe will begin to work for you, at least to some degree. This will give you the evidence you need, the certainty that you have MBS, and the confidence to go forward in your recovery.

The program is detailed and comprehensive. It will guide you in a step-by-step process of removing the barriers to getting better. However, please remember that you don't have to complete every exercise. There are many tools to use, but you can figure out which ones are most important for you. You may not need to do much (or any) of some of the exercises, such as the emotional processing components. Don't think that you need to do every single exercise in order to recover. Do not hold yourself to a specific time frame for completing them. Hold onto the knowledge that you will recover, but do not worry about how long it will take, even though that is probably foremost in your mind right now. Don't put pressure on yourself to get better right away. I'm hoping that you can trust the process that is in these pages and be patient as you go through them. You will get better! I expect that three things will happen for you by taking this course. First, you will learn to understand yourself much better. Second, you will see significant improvement or cure of your physical symptoms. Finally, you will gain more mastery and control over your emotions and your life.

Components of the Program

The program consists of six "Rs" for curing MBS. These are reading about MBS, repudiation of the physical explanations for your symptoms, writing exercises, reflecting with meditative exercises, reprogramming your mind, and rebuilding your life. This edition also includes a new component, verbal expression of deep emotions, as described below. You have already taken the first step, reading or learning enough about MBS so that you are convinced that you do have MBS and that you can be helped by this program.

The second step is actively rejecting any diagnoses for symptoms actually caused by MBS that you may have been given by doctors who are unfamiliar with MBS. It is very important to take this step. You must have a clear understanding that your back pain is not caused by a bulging disc or spinal stenosis; that your abdominal pain is not caused by irritable bowel syndrome; that your headaches are not caused by migraines; that your whole-body pain is not caused by fibromyalgia; that your jaw pain is not caused by TMJ syndrome. You should understand that your anxiety or depression is not due to a chemical imbalance in your brain or that it is your genetic fate to feel these feelings. Even though these diagnoses may help to explain your symptoms and validate them as "real," they are not helpful in terms of curing your symptoms. Of course, I am not asking you to repudiate physical disorders such as hypothyroidism, rheumatoid arthritis, cancer, or heart disease.

It is absolutely true that your symptoms are real; they are not imagined or just in your head. In fact, anyone who says that your symptoms are "all in your head" is ignorant that all pain (and all symptoms) are produced in the brain. What they often imply is that the pain/symptoms are not real, that you are imagining them, that they are your fault, and even that you "want" to have them. Nothing could be further from the truth. I have had MBS symptoms at many points in my life and I can assure you that they are very real! The symptoms are in the mind and body, are caused by a set of learned neural circuits that have been activated, and are caused by Mind Body Syndrome. I have found that it is critical to be able to state clearly and forcefully, "I have Mind Body Syndrome, and I can cure myself (or "I have a neural circuit condition" or "this is my brain and I can cure myself"). This is always the first thing that I do. I ask this question: What is wrong with you? If my patient can say, "nothing," then I am confident that they are ready to move into the treatment phase of the program. It is a powerful statement that repudiates any of the diagnoses that doctors have made that may have caused fear and concern of physical damage.

Some people have doubts about saying that there is nothing wrong with them. They may harbor some doubt that there is a physical cause for their symptoms. In this case, please review chapter five, especially the FIT criteria, to make sure that you are on the right track here. It is normal to have doubts that you will actually recover, as everyone wonders about that. But the question here is "What is wrong with you?" And, if you do have MBS, the correct answer is "Nothing!" There is nothing physically wrong, i.e., no tissue damage and I would add that there is nothing mentally wrong either. You have activated neural circuits that are reversible, that's it.

For the first exercise in this program, I invite you to do the following. Repeat the following sentence to yourself silently. "I have Mind Body Syndrome, and I can cure myself." Now repeat it to yourself out loud. Now do it more loudly and forcefully. Say it again with determination and belief that you will get better. Say it with a smile on your face, knowing that you are on the road to getting better. Say it to members of your family, to your friends, to anyone who is a support for you. There should be no shame in saying this, because you understand that everyone has MBS to some degree at some time in their life. As I've mentioned, I have had it, and I continue to get MBS symptoms at times now in response to emotions or sometimes with no obvious provocation or stressful situation. That is our human condition; that is how our minds and bodies were made. The more you are able to be open with yourself and others about MBS, and the more you are able to accept the diagnosis as the true underlying source of your symptoms, the quicker you will be able to get better.

One of the most difficult things to understand about MBS is that the symptoms can be very severe. It is extremely difficult for people with severe pain, anxiety, depression, or fatigue to grasp the idea that their condition is not caused by some kind of severe physical damage or injury. As I have mentioned, once a serious medical or psychiatric problem is ruled out, you can assume that the problem is MBS. It is surprising but true that MBS can cause very severe symptoms. Many of my patients say things like this: "I can't believe that pain or anxiety this severe can be caused by my brain" and "It's hard to imagine that things that you are not aware of (what's going on the subconscious mind) can have that much power over you." Yet it is true.

Consider the role that pain plays as a protective mechanism. As I have mentioned, if one of our ancestors was running across the savanna and breaks an ankle, it is necessary for his or her brain to generate pain that is severe enough to make him or her stop running and rest, in order to heal and recover. This mechanism has been in place in our brain for many centuries. Since emotions and stress activate the exact same mechanisms as does a physical injury, we often get very severe pain. The brain is attempting to tell us that we are in danger to protect us. It's just that in the case of MBS, the danger is not a physical injury, but rather some kind of social situation that our brain has decided is "dangerous." Therefore, do not be fooled by how severe or how frequent your symptoms are. The pain or other symptoms are not imaginary or simply "in your head." Your brain has learned them, and you can reverse them.

While it can be quite difficult to believe that our minds can cause severe pain, it is often even more difficult to imagine that our minds can cause other symptoms, such as itching, burning, tingling, numbness, fatigue, anxiety, depression, or insomnia. In fact, people who have the most severe, unusual, and widespread symptoms are most likely to have MBS. The purpose of the symptoms is to alert us to do something. When we figure out that certain symptoms are really MBS, the mind often creates new symptoms (or resurrects old ones). Sometimes, the symptom that is created is a form of obsessive-compulsive disorder, thoughts with specific patterns. You might begin to worry about the symptoms, wonder if there is something physically wrong, worry that the doctors missed something, doubt the diagnosis of MBS, or just focus on the symptoms virtually all the time. Understand that these obsessive thoughts are a form of MBS, our minds creating more fear. All of the symptoms of MBS, including the unusual ones and the obsessive thoughts, can be effectively treated when you are clear that you are not damaged, that you need to take control of fear in order to refuse to give them power over you.

Why does this program work so well? The reason we see such rapid and complete responses is that the program addresses the underlying cause of MBS, which is the painful neural circuits that have been learned by the brain and the body. When you repeat the sentence "I have MBS and I can cure myself," you are calming the danger/alarm mechanism of the brain. You are using your conscious mind to affect the subconscious circuits that have been activated and have become persistent. Since there is nothing physically wrong with you, lowering the danger signal is all you need to do to recover. The rest of the program does the same thing. The writing, reflecting, reprogramming, and rebuilding exercises are all designed to activate the conscious portions of the brain to help you unlearn your pain.

Studies by Kirsch (1985) and Bandura (1997) have demonstrated that people who expect that they will improve and those who believe that they have the ability to master their situations (known as self-efficacy) are much more likely to get better. I believe that each and every person with Mind Body Syndrome can get better because it is possible to overcome MBS by using this program. Those people who are unable to accept that their symptoms are due to MBS, or who do not develop positive expectations of relief, or who are unable to believe that they can make changes in their health and in their lives are the people who are less likely to improve.

While some people are able to quickly reverse MBS, it is more common that it takes several weeks to months. It can be frustrating to read about some of the rapid recovery stories described in this and other books. Please be patient and recognize that the neural circuits of MBS may have been activated for quite some time and therefore it can take time to unlearn them. These circuits are like habits that have built up over time and making new habits is often a slow and gradual process. If you put too much pressure on yourself to get better quickly, if you feel that you have to do each and every exercise completely and perfectly, if you want to get better so much that you can't stand to wait for these neural pathways to reverse, you will tend to undermine your progress. I know how hard this can be, as I have gone through it myself, but you can do it. Unlearning Mind Body Syndrome is like training a puppy: it takes a consistent message, persistence over time knowing that the course will have its ups and downs, and doing it with a caring, loving attitude towards yourself.

A Commitment to Heal

I urge you to do this program wholeheartedly and diligently. However, there are a few caveats. As I mentioned above, you can do this program at your own pace. If it takes you more than four weeks, that is perfectly fine. Feel free to decide what is best for you. Taking on a large commitment at a time when you are extremely busy can be stressful in itself, and my intention is not to add more stress to your life. As I noted in chapter 4, many people who have MBS are high achievers or perfectionists. They are likely to be hard on themselves and "beat themselves up" for not reaching their goals. Do not fall into the trap of working too hard on this program, and do not get down on yourself if you miss doing the homework on one or more days. You will have success in this program, but don't create unnecessary worry by putting too much pressure on yourself.

The most important single piece of advice that I can give you is: Be kind to yourself. There are enough stressors in the world and in your life. Don't put more pressure on yourself. Don't increase your guilt or self-blame or self-criticism. These are factors that create MBS and can prevent its cure. Take it easy on yourself. Don't beat yourself up. Don't worry if you don't see improvements immediately. Continue to do the exercises in this program. If you do, you will benefit, and the people in your life will benefit. Most people with MBS do not take enough time for themselves and don't do enough for themselves. Finally, understand that you are going to get better. It may take time, but you will. Even though this program is designed for 28 days, it is often just the beginning of a journey of recovery. If you know that you will get better and that it could take a month or several months or a year, you would probably be fine with that. Everyone is different and while some people rid themselves of pain in a short time, in others, it just takes longer. You may need help along the way, but you will get there.

In summary, it is critical that you believe that you have MBS and that you can be cured. It is critical that you take the time to do the program wholeheartedly. And it is critical to be kind to yourself as you take this time to improve your health and your life.

chapter 7

Week One: Taking Control of Your Life

I have much ado to know myself. — William Shakespeare

I need to move, I need to wake up, I need to change, I need to shake up.
I need to speak out, something's got to break up, I've been asleep, and
I need to wake up. Now. — Melissa Etheridge

Anger is an acid that can do more harm to the vessel in which it is
stored than to anything on which it is poured. — Mark Twain

During the first week, you will learn important skills that you will use during the rest of the program. You will have these skills for the rest of your life. This chapter will introduce you to the exercises that are the basis of the MBS program, which include written and verbal expression, reflection, and reprogramming the mind. If you are new to this work and you are completing the full program, you can set aside up to an hour a day. However, not everyone needs to do that. There are many tools in the book and I suggest that you pick and choose which ones fit your needs. The time you take for yourself will change your life. The next four chapters are packed with a great deal of information to help you in your recovery. I suggest you review the contents of each chapter before starting the exercises to get a sense of what you will be doing. The program entails two different exercises each day, such as a meditation in the morning and a writing exercise in the evening. In addition, the "reprogramming the brain" exercises are meant to be used many times during the day, depending on your situation. Find out for yourself which exercises are most helpful to you and practice them at your own pace. Don't pressure yourself to do every exercise or to recover within a certain time frame; doing so can delay recovery. Know that you will recover. Relax and proceed at your own pace.

Reprogramming the Brain

As you are now aware, your brain has developed neural circuits that are causing your MBS symptoms. These circuits are real and have developed because of the stressful events in your life, the (often subconscious) emotions that were generated by these events, and the internal pressures that you put on yourself. These circuits that have created pain and other symptoms are learned and can be unlearned. This section introduces you to one of the most important and useful components of the program.

For you to cure MBS, the neural circuits that continue to produce pain or other MBS symptoms need to be interrupted. Fortunately, you do not have to undo these circuits nor do you have to create new circuits to take their place. You still have the normal circuits for the times when you were not in pain, not feeling anxious or depressed or fatigued. You will be reactivating these circuits as you deactivate the circuits causing your symptoms. Many of you have probably seen that your symptoms can come and go, sometimes very quickly; or that the symptoms shift from one location to another; or that they have changed over time. Symptoms that are in identical spots on both sides of the body in a symmetric fashion are also often MBS, as the brain easily creates those types of symptoms. Symptoms of tingling, burning, numbness are often MBS as well. Symptoms that radiate from one side of the body to another, up and down one side of the body, or involve the whole leg or arm are typical of MBS. All these phenomena are evidence that the symptoms are coming from neural circuits that are changeable. Pain that is constant and never varies or moves can also be MBS. As long as there is not a clearly identifiable cause based upon your medical evaluation, this type of pain is also highly likely to be MBS. The research on the causes of pain support this. Of the people with chronic pain, very few actually have an ongoing structural cause for their pain; and this ncludes people with headaches, abdominal and pelvic pain, arm and leg pain, neck and back pain, and widespread pain syndromes.

Research studies show that when you change how you think or how you react to stressful situations, you are actually changing your brain and its circuits (Doidge, 2007; Begley, 2008). In fact, the brain is constantly changing and developing new circuits. That is why studies have shown that people with chronic pain and fatigue have changes that can be seen in the brain (May, 2008; Baliki, et. al., 2008; Lange, et. al., 1999). While some researchers believe that these changes are evidence that chronic pain and fatigue are actually disease states of the brain, it seems more likely that these changes are caused by the symptoms. When one learns and practices a new skill of any kind, such as playing an instrument or a new video game, the brain is changed. Similarly, "learned" pain is also "practiced" when the pain persists for some time and it makes perfect sense that these changes will be visualized by sophisticated brain imaging techniques. It has been shown that the brain also changes with therapy and the resolution of psychological symptoms, as has been demonstrated in people with spider phobias (Paquette, et. al., 2003). When people with several years of chronic pain get better and resolve their symptoms, they are proving that the brain can change even after it has learned and practiced pain. Exercises that reprogram the mind teach you to activate the conscious part of the brain to override the subconscious pathways that produce and maintain pain and MBS. When you practice these exercises, you are changing your brain. The more you practice, the quicker you will get better. Studies of people who have had strokes show that they can rewire their brains (Taub, et. al., 2006). With enough practice, they relearn how to use their limbs that were paralyzed. This usually takes a great deal of time and practice. A similar process occurs in people with closed head injuries or traumatic brain injuries (TBI). These injuries affect the brain temporarily, often with dizziness, nausea, and other symptoms. However, the brain will rewire itself to heal. In some people, they may develop persistent symptoms of TBI, such as memory loss, brain fog, fatigue, eye issues and other symptoms. It is likely that these ongoing symptoms are actually due to MBS after some time has occurred for brain healing. These neural circuits can be unlearned using this program. Fortunately, reprogramming the brain to unlearn MBS usually takes less time than recovering from a stroke. However, everyone is different, so don't worry if you don't see changes immediately. It may be necessary to repeat the following exercises for several weeks or months until your brain responds by re-activating the symptom-free circuits that are still present from the time before you had MBS.

Many people with chronic pain or other symptoms are plagued by the concern that there is a physical cause for their symptoms. They find it hard to believe that their brain and its neural circuits ways could produce so much pain. But pain that comes and goes or that moves to different places within the body is clearly caused by neural pathways. However, constant pain or other symptoms that occur consistently with certain movements or positions can also be MBS. If this is true for you, pay closer attention to see if your brain offers you some clues. A patient of mine had pain in his left heel that seemed to be coming from a structural cause. It hurt each time he walked on it, and it was tender when he pushed against it. However, one time he woke during the night and walked to the bathroom and back to bed with no pain at all. The next day, after he recalled this, he began to walk with confidence that the pain in his heel was, in fact, MBS. This was a turning point in his recovery. If pain occurs when you sit in certain chairs but not others, this is a typical sign that you're dealing with MBS. When symptoms increase, pay attention to see if there was some trigger, such as an event or a thought that created fear, resentment, guilt, or sadness. At times, an increase in symptoms will occur for no apparent reason because neural circuits that produce the pain have not yet been reversed. If you continue to investigate symptoms, your brain will usually give you clues that the symptoms are due to MBS. Understanding that message will give you more confidence in turning these symptoms around.

Reprogramming MBS Symptoms: Pain Reprocessing Therapy (PRT)

Pain reprocessing therapy is a term we use for reprogramming or rewiring the neural circuits in the brain. The term was coined by my colleague, Alan Gordon, LCSW, who developed many of these techniques. PRT includes a range of attitudes and exercises that we have found extremely useful in reversing chronic pain and other symptoms caused by MBS. We studied this method in a randomized, controlled research study that we call the Boulder back pain study (Ashar, 2022). In this trial, we randomized 150 people in Boulder, Colorado who had chronic back pain for approximately 10 years in duration. A third of them had a placebo back injection, a third had treatment as usual (no specific intervention), and a third got PRT. I personally evaluated 45 of the 50 who were randomized to the PRT arm of the study (5 dropped out) and I determined that 43 of the 45 had MBS, i.e., no structural cause for their back pain, based upon the criteria described in chapter 5 of this book. Of those who were treated, 75% of them were pain free in one month; an amazing result, which is much better than the outcomes for chronic back pain in other traditional treatment programs. You can find out more about PRT in The Way Out (Gordon and Ziv, 2021). Another research study done at Harvard by Michael Donnino also showed that this approach led to 64% of the patients with chronic back pain becoming pain-free (Donnino, 2021).

MBS is caused by neural circuits that become persistent due to four main factors: 1) natural reactions to pain and other symptoms, 2) ongoing emotional reactions to past and current stressful life situations, 3) personality traits that we have discussed, and 4) ongoing stressful situations that need correcting or adapting to. PRT focuses on addressing the first of these, our natural reactions to pain and other symptoms. When the brain generates pain, it looks for feedback to determine whether to make this pain persistent (keep those neural circuits activated) or turn off the pain. The brain looks for input from the nerves coming into the brain from the body to see if there is ongoing tissue damage, which fortunately is absent in MBS. The brain considers our past experiences with pain and injury as well as our past experiences with stress and trauma, which we will address later. A critical input to the brain is how we respond to the symptom itself.

Most people will respond to pain, especially severe pain and chronic pain, with alarm. Of course, that is the purpose of pain: to generate alarm and concern, in order to act to create a safe environment for healing. When pain occurs due to physical injury, we appropriately react by stopping activities, avoiding any other injury, and getting help. Our natural reactions consist of what I call the six Fs:

Fear of the pain or other symptom: We fear the sensation of it as it can be so severe and unpleasant; we worry about whether it will go away and when or when it will return; we spend a lot of time wishing it will go away

Fous on the pain or other symptom: We pay a lot of attention to it; we monitor it; we focus on how it feels and if it is changing or getting worse

Frustration with it: We get upset, annoyed and angry at the pain or other symptom; we become resentful that doctors haven't fixed it or don't understand it; we become sad for what we have lost

Fighting it: We work hard to overcome it; we try to push through it; and we get exhausted in the fight, especially when we feel we are losing the battle

Trying to figure it out: We spend a lot of time thinking about it; we search for answers online, in doctor's offices and with alternative care practices

Trying to fix it: We spend a lot of time and money on treatments that haven't worked; we try anything and everything that might work; we get desperate for a cure; we get depressed when one doesn't materialize

Everyone engages in most of these reactions, which are very helpful when there is a structural condition causing pain or other symptoms. However, when the diagnosis is MBS, these are exactly the reactions that you do NOT want to engage in. These reactions send feedback to the brain that "Yes, there is a problem; a big problem." This feedback makes the brain continue to generate pain and actually make it worse over time. This is the vicious cycle we call the Pain-Fear-Pain cycle for short. The following diagram explains the neural circuitry of MBS.

Pain Reprocessing Therapy addresses the six Fs and teaches us how to provide corrective feedback to the brain's danger mechanism in order to guide the brain towards turning off the pain or other symptoms. It interrupts the vicious cycle of pain to provide lasting relief. I often use this analogy with patients. When a child falls off of a bicycle, often they immediately look to the adult to figure out if they should cry or not. If the adult shows fear, they will cry; but if the adult smiles and says: "You're OK, that was something," they may not cry. We will teach you to give your brain feedback that it's OK, and that you are OK.

It is important to understand that the brain is not trying to betray you or hurt you. It is doing

Pain Circuitry Becomes the Neural Circuitry of MBS

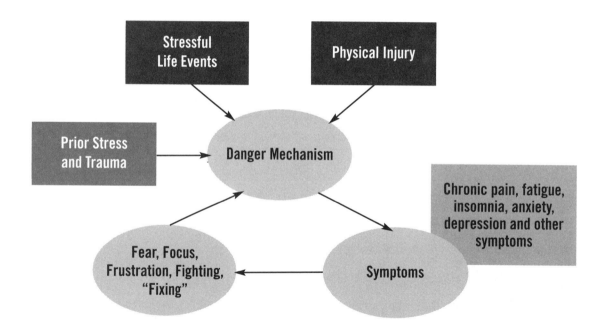

THE NEURAL CIRCUITS THAT PRODUCE AND PERPETUATE MIND BODY SYNDROME: The danger mechanism in the brain can be activated by physical injury or by stressful life situations, or a combination of the two. In MBS, there is no ongoing physical injury. The neural circuits of danger create pain and other MBS symptoms as an alarm. Natural reactions to these symptoms of the six Fs send feedback to the brain that leads to persistent and increasing pain over time. The danger mechanism can also be sensitized to activate the danger signal by prior life stresses and traumatic life events.

its job to the best of its ability. It is trying to protect you by sending a message that something is wrong. Your brain can't tap you on the shoulder and say: "By the way, my friend, what you're going through is just horrible or wrong, and I'm sounding an alarm to let you know this." The danger signal is like a smoke alarm. And we don't get angry with a smoke alarm; it is just doing its job. We don't know why the brain chooses to produce certain symptoms as opposed to others at a given time nor do we know why the brain is wired to produce pain when both physical injury or emotional injury occurs, but it clearly does. I often use this analogy to describe how we can respond to the brain when it generates pain or other symptoms: Think of a child lying in bed, fearful of a monster in the closet. Would you be angry at this child? Of course, not. You put aside your annoyance at being woken up or called, you open the closet door to show them that there is no monster there, you lie down with the child and calm them, soothe them with compassion and caring, and then tell them a story. That is exactly what you need to do to calm the danger signal so that the brain turns off the pain or other symptoms. You will gently tell your brain that there is no tissue damage here, you are OK, and you can do this with kindness, not anger. You will thank the brain for sounding the alarm, as you know it is just trying to protect you and help you. You will calm the brain by telling it there's nothing wrong physically and that you will be able to handle the stress that is occurring or that did occur in the past. You will smile and go on with your day. You can know that by doing this you are gradually turning down the danger mechanism and training the brain out of pain.

EXERCISE 1: THE QUIZ AND AFFIRMATIONS

As you begin this work to rewire the neural circuits in your brain, there will be several exercises for you to do on a regular basis. These exercises are very simple and straightforward. In fact, they may seem too simple or silly to do any good, especially in the face of severe pain or other symptoms. However, they do work. We know this and we see this every day with our patients. Just as with the fallen or fearful child, we just need to soothe the brain and the best ways to do that are with the truth (that nothing is actually wrong), with humor and a smile, and with kindness.

Go back to the quiz from the last chapter. Ask yourself this question: "What's wrong with you?" And then answer yourself: "NOTHING IS WRONG!" Remember that this is the truth and that this truth will set you free. If you have doubts about this, review the FIT criteria from chapter 5 or seek more help and advice. If you are sure though, go ahead and answer this quiz with a smile, with gusto, with laughter and relief, knowing that you are going to get better. You can sing this to yourself, you can do this in another language, or in a funny accent. All of these may seem silly, but they are powerful ways of calming your brain. Take this quiz several times a day as you start this program.

In addition to taking this quiz for yourself, create a set of affirmations for yourself. If you thought that the quiz was silly, this may sound even worse! I always thought that affirmations were kind of stupid, but there is sound research showing that they are effective and they do change the brain (Cascio, 2016).

Here are a set of affirmations that I commonly recommend, but please make up your own set and make them yours. Again, you can sing them, whisper them, shout them, laugh with them, do them in different languages and accents.

I'm healthy

I'm strong

There is absolutely nothing wrong with me

I'm not afraid

I'm in charge, I can do what I want

I'm safe, I'm not in danger, I'll be fine.

You can do these affirmations several times a day at the beginning, but you will not be doing them the rest of your life! You can do them while walking, driving, or doing chores or anytime you can find a few moments. Another twist on this is to do the affirmations while standing up in a position of "power."

Positions of power are expansive, i.e., ones in which you stand, inhale deeply, put your arms up or put your hands on our hips, and move your feet apart to the width of your shoulders. This type of body position leads to changes in your physiology, resulting in increases in testosterone (a power hormone), decreases in cortisol (a stress hormone), and increases in the pain threshold (leading to decreased pain) (Choi, et. al., 2012; Bohns, et. al., 2012). People who assume this type of powerful position for a couple of minutes do better on tests and job interviews than those in submissive positions, such as being curled up in a ball or sitting with head in hands (Carney, et. al., 2010). If you are so inclined, I even give you permission to use curse words as part of your affirmations. In fact, research shows that using swear words can reduce pain (Stephens, 2009; Stephens and Umland, 2011).

Remember that as you do these exercises, your goal is to reduce the fear of pain and to reduce the other natural reactions (the "six Fs"). Your goal is not to reduce the pain. This may seem odd to you. Of course, you want to reduce the pain and other symptoms. But the way to get to those reductions is by calming the brain. You do not have direct control over the danger signal in your brain. It will do what it wants for a while. You do have control over how you respond to the symptoms and how you relate to them. Each time you take the quiz, each time you do your affirmations and each time you do the other exercises in this program, you are investing in calming the danger signal. You are training your brain out of pain, and out of anxiety and depression as well. Your brain will get the message. You will get better.

Many people are faced with constant pain, and they could spend their whole day talking to their mind and their body. In this situation, you will need to practice this exercise very frequently, but certainly not all day. It is not a good idea to focus on the pain or other symptoms. The more you pay attention to pain, anxiety, fatigue, and depression, the worse it tends to get. Three studies on pain have confirmed this. People who were instructed to keep a "pain diary" to monitor and track their frequency and level of pain had large increases in pain, in comparison to those who did not keep such pain diaries (Ferrari, et. al., 2010; Ferrari, et. al., 2013; Ferrari, 2015). The more you can focus on living your life while using the affirmations above and the less time you focus on the symptoms, the quicker you will recover.

One of my colleagues, Alan Gordon, MFT, describes this phenomenon very well. He notes that every time you think about your pain, feel frustration over it, monitor it, hate it, or feel despair over it, you are being preoccupied by it, wondering how much or when it's going to hurt. The same can be true for anxiety, depression, fatigue, or other MBS symptoms. Your mind is a relentless machine, churning out thought after thought and fear after fear about your symptoms.

One of the most powerful ways to overcome MBS is by training yourself to be completely indifferent to the symptoms. This can be very hard but with practice you can do this. Begin to notice how you respond to pain or other MBS symptoms. Most people react with disappointment, fear, or hopelessness. These natural responses make the symptoms more likely to persist. Try new responses to your symptoms. Tell yourself: "I know what you are (MBS), and I know that you are trying to lead me to disappointment, fear, and hopelessness. However, I will not go there. I am safe and getting better. I am fine, and I will be fine." One of my teenaged patients found it helpful to simply press an imaginary "delete" button when she noticed the fear. This shortcut shifted her brain towards something else. An adult patient of mine would treat the fear as if it were a solicitation phone call and just "hang up."

Begin to practice this and be proud of yourself for responding in such a healthy way. Then take some deep breaths to help calm you down and move on to focus on something else in your life. Even if you don't see results initially, keep practicing—it may take some time to retrain the brain.

EXERCISE 2: MINDFUL AWARENESS/SOMATIC TRACKING

This exercise offers another method for changing your relationship with your pain, anxiety, or other symptoms. This is a type of a meditative process that consists of sitting still and observing the sensations occurring in your body from moment to moment. It is very similar to mindfulness meditation, which many of you have done. However, there are a couple of key differences that make it particularly applicable to reducing MBS. When one pays attention to physical sensations, such as pain, anxiety or fatigue, they do not necessarily improve, especially when the sensations are considered to be due to some kind of a structural or physical problem. This program helps people to re-categorize their physical sensations as being due to MBS. This is a critical difference. When one knows that the sensations are MBS, that there is no physical damage, that the sensations are essentially harmless, and that they will get better, then it is much, much easier to pay attention to them without fear or worry, to separate from them, to simply observe them as "just sensations" or even as "just thoughts." In my experience, this makes all the difference.

Before beginning this process, there is a preliminary exercise that makes it more effective. I borrowed this technique from the Internal Family Systems approach (Schwartz and Sweezy, 2020).

Sit in a comfortable position. Take a few soft, slow breaths. Think about the symptom you have, whether it's pain, anxiety, insomnia, fatigue or any other MBS symptom. Ask yourself this question: How do I feel towards this symptom or sensation? Do I fear it? Do I hate it? Am I annoyed by it, resentful of it? Worried about it? Feel guilty about it? Or all of the above?

Identify these feelings within you. See if you can be aware of each of them separately. Some people actually can visualize the feelings. Then gently ask that feeling to "step aside" for a few moments or gently "reach inside" of yourself and place the feeling outside of you, on a table or chair for a few moments. You are not trying to completely get rid of the anger or the fear towards your symptom, you are just setting it aside for a bit. You can let the anger or fear subside for now. You don't need or want it for this mindful awareness/somatic tracking exercise. See how it feels to let go of resentment or worry towards your pain or other symptoms for now. It might feel like a relief.

As mentioned, the mindful awareness/somatic tracking process consists of sitting in silence and observing the sensations that arise on a moment by moment basis. The key to this exercise is to recognize is that your body is not damaged and that the sensations you are currently feeling are generated by your brain. However, even if you have some doubts about this, you will still be able to do this exercise. It usually provides a great deal of insight into your situation. The recorded meditation Mindful Awareness/Somatic Tracking exercise is available at unlearnyourpain.com, under the Meditations menu at the top of the home page; the password is: meditations

A synoposis of the meditation is provided on the following page. The goal is to sit and observe sensations as they arise. Since these sensations are created by the brain, there is no immediate danger to you. Therefore, you can practice watching these sensations, even if they are quite painful or uncomfortable, without as much reaction or fear. Through this process, you will learn to tolerate these sensations more and more. As you do this, you are showing your brain that these sensations are not dangerous and don't need to be feared. This process turns down the danger/alarm mechanism and the fear response of the brain, which in turn, reduces pain, anxiety and other symptoms.

As you practice this meditation of observing without fear, you will often note that the sensations you will feel will shift over time. Often, this occurs within a few minutes. Painful or anxious sensations will lessen or increase or move to different parts of the body. All of these changes are evidence that the brain is actually generating and altering these sensations. This becomes more proof that you have MBS. If you continue to watch and remind yourself that these sensations are not evidence of a physical disorder, you can take the attitude that it doesn't matter if they get better, get worse, or go away. You are just watching the process. You can smile as you watch the "show" that your brain is putting on for you. When you do that, you are training yourself to tolerate these symptoms and reduce fear, which furthers your recovery.

As you do this exercise, you will often find that many different thoughts, feelings and physical sensations occur. This is part of the normal activity of the brain as it produces a variety of mental and physical phenomena. Use this exercise to observe your brain in action. You will see that it creates physical sensations, thoughts that range from simple to silly to very fearful, feelings such as sadness, guilt or anger, anxiety or tension, and periods of calm. This exercise is designed to see all of this clearly and treat all of these mental products the same: meeting them with calm, ease, understanding, and kindness, even if (especially if) they create fear and worry within you. As you face these sensations, you can breathe into them and gradually train yourself to face them, tolerate them and detach from them. As you do that, they will tend to shift over time, from one to the other and back again. Just keep watching and observing, knowing that this is your brain in action and that these sensations are creations of the brain that cannot hurt you or harm you. You are in the process of changing the neural circuits in your brain by reducing the danger/alarm mechanism. And over time, you will see how these sensations shift and gain evidence that all of these are, in fact, caused by the brain and that you are not damaged or broken. You are on the path to recovery.

Mindful Awareness Synopsis

Sit in a comfortable position. Turn your attention to the breath. Notice the breath without needing to change it. Paying attention to the details, knowing there is nothing wrong with your breathing, just watching the breath and seeing how and if it shifts over time. Watch your breath as you would watch clouds in the sky. And adding a touch of kindness as you observe the breath.

Turn your attention to any feelings of anxiety or discomfort. Noticing these sensations without needing to change them or alter them. Paying attention to the details, knowing that there is nothing wrong in the body, that the brain is causing these sensations. Continuing to just watch these sensations, without fearing them. Seeing if and how they shift over time, not caring if the sensations get better, get worse, stay the same or go away. It doesn't matter, just observing them as if watching clouds, knowing that you are safe and not in danger. Noticing any sensations without any fear, worries or concerns.

When the sensations shift in any way, then turning your attention to the new or different sensation. Once again, noticing without any need to change them. Paying attention to the details and allowing yourself to feel these sensations without fear. They can't hurt or harm you. Knowing there is nothing wrong in the body, that the brain is causing these sensations. Continue to observe the sensations, without fearing them. Seeing if and how they shift over time. Adding a touch of kindness. Knowing that you are safe and not in danger. Watching without fear, worry or concern. Not caring if the sensations get better or worse or even change, it doesn't matter. Observing as if watching clouds in the sky. Seeing if you can allow yourself to feel these sensations as less unpleasant than you have in the past.

Finishing the exercise by returning your attention to the breathing. Breathe in kindness to yourself, breathe in strength, breathe in calmness.

Repeat this exercise several times a day, especially when you notice anxiety or physical symptoms, but also at other times to practice reducing fear and learning to separate from symptoms that are caused by the brain.

EXERCISE 3: NEURAL CIRCUIT TESTING

This exercise offers a way to learn more about how your brain may be generating symptoms and how to reverse the process. Research has shown that when someone imagines having an injury, the brain activates areas that are identical to when there is an actual injury (Derbyshire, 2004). We can use this process to demonstrate how your brain may be working by asking you to imagine certain scenarios.

Most people with chronic pain and other symptoms have particular things that trigger these symptoms. Do you remember that man who sustained a shrapnel wound in the Viet Nam war? He would get pain in the area of his original injury years later when he heard the sound of a helicopter. The helicopter was his trigger. It triggered his brain to activate a particular neural circuit of pain. His brain learned that association, just as did Pavlov's dogs learned the association between the buzzer he rang and food, thus causing them to salivate when they heard the buzzer. This happens to most people and often there is no clear reason why the brain might have developed that association, but it does. I have seen many people who developed pain with certain movements, when they visit certain places, when they are exposed to hot or cold water, certain foods or sounds or smells. Weather is a common trigger as well as computer screens or typing. Many people react to either light or deeper touch or pressure in certain spots. Once the brain learns this neural association, it often becomes persistent and can spread over time. People who started out thinking that they had an allergy to one food or one chemical, begin to have similar reactions to other foods, and this can spiral out of control. The brain begins to react to these triggers as dangers and activates circuits of pain or other symptoms. On the other hand, when the brain reacts to certain stimuli or situations as being "safe," the brain turns off the symptoms. We see this with massages, acupuncture, herbal products or supplements, Reiki, hot baths or certain exercises. Once you recognize which triggers are activating your brain's danger signal, you can work to move those triggers into the category of safe activities. This exercise will teach you how to do that.

Make a list of your triggers. Include things such as light, sounds, smells, foods, chemical, weather patterns, screens, typing, certain movements or positions, exercises, touch or deeper pressure, certain people, places, situations or anything else.

_____

_____

_____

_____

_____

_____

_____

_____

_____

_____

_____

Step One:

Close your eyes and sit in a comfortable position. Or assume a position that would fit for the trigger, such as standing up if the trigger is bending forward or sitting down. Imagine that you are engaging in one of the triggering activities from your list right now. Picture yourself doing the activity or being in the situation as vividly as you can.

See what reaction occurs. Do you get pain with this imagination? Or anxiety? Or some muscle tension? Or even an emotional reaction? Or did you get no reaction at all. Either way is fine.

If you get some kind of reaction, even if it's a small one, this is showing you that your brain is sensitized to this trigger and is activating your symptoms. This is important information for you and shows the power of the brain to create these sensations. Now, calm your brain in relation to the feelings in your body when you imagine this activity. You can smile at your brain. Breathe slowly. Know that this reaction is caused by your brain and you are OK. Allow the sensations to subside.

If no reaction occurs, that's fine too. This just shows that your brain isn't quite that sensitized. You still do have MBS though, which you confirmed by doing the exercises in chapter 5.

Step Two:

Now you can proceed to the next step. Smile, and tell yourself that you are fine, healthy, strong, not in danger, safe and not afraid, i.e., repeat the set of affirmations you have developed.

Then imagine doing that activity again, but this time, imagine you are engaged in this activity with joy and ease in your heart and in your mind. Imagine how good this will feel to engage in this activity without any fear or worry.

See what reaction you get this time.

Continue imagining that activity without fear and with joy and ease in your heart and mind, until you can imagine doing it with that attitude and until you get no sensations at all in your body, except for a good feeling of accomplishment and happiness.

Step Three:

Then, when you are beginning to develop some confidence, take this same attitude of fearlessness, joy and ease and engage in the activity in a very small way. This may be sitting for only a few seconds without fear, or bending over slowly once, or walking a block, or just looking at certain foods or taking a tiny bite of it, or typing a few words, or driving to a certain place but not even going in, or pressing lightly on a tender spot on your body. As long as you do this activity with your affirmations, with certainty you are fine and will be fine, and with a smile, you are training your brain out of MBS. It doesn't matter if you get any symptoms or not.

Continue doing that until you can do this small amount of exposure to the trigger without any symptoms, or with minimal symptoms that you can reassure yourself are not important as they are just coming from your brain and nothing is wrong with you. You can even look forward to getting some symptoms, as this is your time to practice and reprogram your brain.

Step Four:

Gradually, begin to do more over time. Expose your brain to more of the trigger, while continuing to remind your brain that everything is OK. Recognize that your brain may create no symptoms one day, and then for no reason at all, create increased symptoms the next day. Do not worry about that. You can expect that to happen. It is a normal part of the recovery process. But don't stop. Keep going forward and you will gradually rewire the neural circuits of MBS.

Step Five:

Then choose another activity from your list of triggers and start to work on that in the same way. You will gradually unlearn these triggers and you will take large steps towards recovering from MBS. You'll get there. You are going to get better!

For some demonstrations on neural circuit testing, which I also refer to as provocative testing, you can go to unlearnyourpain.com, click on the Media tab at the top of the home page, select videos, and click on neural circuit testing demonstration.

More Information on Triggers

Most people have triggers that tend to activate pain or other symptoms. These are often some activity, but they can also be a certain location, specific thoughts or memories, certain foods or positions, specific times of day, certain seasons or not infrequently anniversaries of significant events. No matter what your triggers are, it is critical to know that these situations, not tissue damage or disease, activate the learned neural pathways in your brain, and those pathways can be unlearned. Most people know how to control their body, like when you tell your brain and bladder not to urinate at an inappropriate time or place. You can alter physical reactions activated by the brain. Practice doing so as often as you can as you start this program.

Most people learn to avoid the triggers that cause pain or other MBS symptoms. While this approach is often recommended by doctors and seems to make common sense, in the long run it is not a good strategy for recovery. The more you avoid these triggers, the greater power they begin to have over you. Avoiding certain foods or locations or positions or activities can create fear and insecurity. Fear and insecurity will create more pain, more anxiety, and the triggers can get worse or spread to new triggers over time. I have seen people who began by avoiding a few foods or chemicals and over time, were unable to tolerate more and more foods or chemicals.

Remember that a trigger is something that turns on the symptom by activating the neural circuit that causes it; it does not cause the symptom by causing tissue damage in your body. This is an important distinction. I would not advise someone with a broken ankle to walk on it; this would cause tissue damage. However, I do advise walking on an ankle with pain due to MBS, all the while reminding yourself that this pain is MBS and that you are going to change the circuits. This process will give you a way to meet your triggers head on and learn to overcome them. The more you practice doing this, the sooner you will improve.

A good method of challenging triggers is to anticipate when the trigger is likely to occur and create a set of mental statements to counteract the trigger. Since the trigger acts by activating neural circuits, you will be creating a different set of neural circuits to replace those. This is the same process used to break a bad habit. In order to stop smoking, you can anticipate the times when you are most likely to smoke and create a different habit to replace the smoking habit. The brain learns this new habit and eventually the smoking habit is extinguished. The same is true for pain or other symptoms caused by MBS. If you believe this can work, commit to learning new habits, and repeat it as many times as needed for the brain to learn. You can replace your old habits with new ones.

It helps to create your own set of affirmations that you say to yourself, either out loud or silently as you confront a trigger situation or whenever you feel pain in a certain position or movement or part of the body. Here are some I've found useful:

"I'm healthy. I'm strong. There's nothing wrong with me. I'm not afraid. I can do this activity without pain, without fear. Even if there is some pain, I will be OK." I am getting better, and I'm proud of doing that for myself. I can relax with that knowledge. I don't have to worry anymore. Everything will be fine. I'm OK. There is no danger here; no worries."

After stating these affirmations, engage in the triggering activity with confidence. If the pain or other MBS symptoms lessen, you're on the path to healing. If they don't change, keep at it and you'll see results over time. Even if the pain gets worse, it is important to be strong, maintain courage and confidence, and continue to challenge your triggers. When symptoms worsen, it is usually because you are afraid. If so, reduce the amount of exercise or movement or exposure to the triggering event and work on the fear. Practice calming your mind and reminding yourself that this is MBS and that you are overcoming it.

Alan Gordon uses the term "outcome independence" to define this method of eliminating MBS symptoms. You are successful when you have challenged your fears, no matter if your pain lessens or not. A good example of this comes from the movie, *Dead Poets Society*. In the film, one of the students has a huge crush on a girl from a nearby school but is terrified to ask her out. Finally, he musters his courage and goes to a party she's attending.   Later that night, he returns to his school with a black eye, beaming with joy. His friends ask him what happened.

"I asked her out," he replies with a huge grin.

"And she said yes?" they ask.

"She said 'No,' and then her boyfriend punched me in the face."

"Then why are you so happy??"

"Because I asked."

He was pleased in spite of the outcome because he overcame his fear.

Think how outcome dependent you tend to be with the pain or other MBS symptoms. If you get these symptoms when you walk or bend or go outside, you may limit these activities because you are paying close attention to how severe the symptoms are. These thoughts and fears feed the pain or other symptoms.

Therefore do not measure your success by whether you have pain or other symptoms or how severe they are. You are successful whenever you engage in the things that have triggered symptoms. You are successful when you do the things that you want to do in your life and do not care if the symptoms lessen. It is common for the symptoms to get worse when you begin confronting your triggers. Your mind will try to hang on to the symptoms and will try harder to scare you into turning back. Don't be fooled. This is actually a good sign; your danger signal tends towards maintaining the old status quo. Keep going; know that you are on the right path, and that you will get better.

At the beginning of these activities, tell yourself, "It doesn't matter how much or little it hurts afterward. What matters is how little I let it affect me; how I refuse to let my mood, my self-perception, my feelings about the future be determined by how much pain I'm in afterward."

It is critical to be proud of what you are doing whether or not you have pain or other MBS symptoms. Be happy that you are doing these activities and challenging your fear and preoccupation with symptoms. You are training yourself to focus on what you are doing to heal (the process), rather than on the results (the outcome); you are winning the battle because you are moving forward, whether you have pain or not.

Challenging triggers often requires a great deal of courage. Everyone has fear of pain and other symptoms. Find the best methods for these challenges. Some people start with baby steps and small increments of exposure to their triggers, while others jump in and do more initially. An excellent method for overcoming triggers is to start with a very small exposure to the trigger, such as just taking one step, sitting for 10 seconds, eating a tiny bit of the food, listening to a quiet sound or seeing a computer screen for only a few seconds. As you create a bit of exposure, you allow the danger signal in the brain to become activated. You may feel anxious or tense, you may get the symptom, or you may not. The next step is to breathe, calm your brain, remind yourself that this trigger is not harmful and won't hurt you. As you calm, you are reducing the danger signal. Then repeat the activity to the same degree or to a slightly increased degree, and see what symptoms arise and calm yourself once again. Keep doing this and gradually increase the amount of time or the amount of the trigger as you begin to be more confident and as you turn off the danger signal in the brain. Find your own pace and level of exposure that suits you, but continue to gradually increase your exposure and challenge yourself to heal. Your brain will be activating healthy circuits and the more you practice the less likely it will be that your brain will switch back to the painful circuits. I have great admiration for people who engage in this work. They are brave souls willing to find their own way to health and recovery. They are breaking the chains of pain, anxiety, depression, and other symptoms as they demonstrate their power and commitment to heal.

A good way to achieve outcome independence is to create a goal of doing a certain amount of exercise or work or something that will challenge a trigger to your symptoms. Then work at doing that amount every day or every other day. If you decide you are going to walk or exercise for just a minute or two, make that your goal and disregard whether this causes symptoms or not. If you achieve the exercise goal, celebrate that victory. Focusing on a goal with outcome independence will take precedent over reducing symptoms, and that will lead to overcoming MBS. Then you can gradually build up to a few minutes and then go longer. As long as you are calming yourself, reducing fear, and reminding yourself that you are healthy, there is nothing wrong and you will get better, you are training your brain out of danger.

When you have found ways to reduce pain and other symptoms, you can repeat that process. Over time, you can develop shortcuts to unlearning the neural pathways associated with the symptoms. I had a patient who found that if she drew a bunch of circles on a piece of paper and then burned the paper, she could make the tension in her neck go away. Over time, she drew fewer circles and eventually just imagined drawing the circles and burning the paper to reduce symptoms. I met a teenager who was diagnosed with postural orthostatic tachycardia syndrome (POTS), which is a form of MBS that produces dizziness when standing up. I taught her how to use a set of positive affirmations to prevent herself from developing the dizziness. Over time, she was able to simply say, "OK" whenever she stood up and not be dizzy.

EXERCISE 4: DURING THE DAY EXERCISE

This exercise can be used as you go about your day. It's designed as a brief way of reminding your brain that you're OK and gradually lowering the danger signal in your brain. Whenever you notice one of your MBS symptoms, you can stop for a moment to calm your brain. You want to replace the natural tendency of going into fear and worry with something like this:

You can smile, take a nice slow breath, and say to yourself:

"That's interesting. That's my brain. This is just a sensation. It's not important and can't harm me. It will pass. I'm OK."

Then take another slow breath and move on with your day.

You don't have to necessarily say all of these each time you notice symptoms. You can choose any shortcuts or other statements. I had a patient who recovered from MBS simply by repeatedly reminding his brain, "I'm OK" during the course of the day. It can also be very effective to speak to yourself in the third person, saying: "You're OK." Or using your name to speak to yourself, or some kind nickname for yourself. Making this work more fun and enjoyable can make all the difference in the world.

Writing Exercise: Addressing Stressor and Personality Traits

List of past traumatic or stressful events: Include any interactions or events which caused hurt, shame, resentment, embarrassment, pain, anger, guilt, humiliation, fear, worry, or other negative emotions. Try to think of anything and everything which falls into this category and list each event or situation as a separate item. Include events from your childhood as far back as you can remember. While you're doing this exercise, put down anything that comes into your mind, even if you are not sure it has a connection to your MBS symptoms.

1. Issue: _____

_____

2. Issue: _____

_____

3. Issue: _____

_____

4. Issue: _____

_____

5. Issue: _____

_____

6. Issue: _____

_____

7. Issue: _____

_____

8. Issue: _____

_____

9. Issue: _____

_____

10. Issue: _____

_____

11. Issue: _____

_____

12. Issue: _____

_____

13. Issue: _____

_____

14. Issue: _____

_____

15. Issue: _____

_____

16. Issue: _____

_____

17. Issue: _____

_____

18. Issue: _____

_____

19. Issue: _____

_____

20. Issue: _____

_____

List of personality traits that may contribute to MBS symptoms: Include traits such as perfectionism, low self-esteem, high expectations of self, worry, fear, anger, hostility, time urgency, guilt, dependency, isolation, needing to be good/liked, being overly conscientious, being hard on yourself, being overly responsible, harboring anger or resentment, not standing up for self and others. Try to think of anything and everything, and list each trait as a separate item. Include personality traits that were learned or developed in childhood as well as those you currently posess.

1. Issue: _____

_____

2. Issue: _____

_____

3. Issue: _____

_____

4. Issue: _____

_____

5. Issue: _____

_____

6. Issue: _____

_____

7. Issue: _____

_____

8. Issue: _____

_____

9. Issue: _____

_____

10. Issue: _____

_____

11. Issue: _____

_____

12. Issue: _____

_____

13. Issue: _____

_____

14. Issue: _____

_____

15. Issue: _____

_____

16. Issue: _____

_____

17. Issue: _____

_____

18. Issue: _____

_____

19. Issue: _____

_____

20. Issue: _____

_____

Writing Away Your Pain

By now, it should be clear that there are two main processes by which MBS begins and becomes persistent: stressful situations in life and learned neural circuits in the brain. This program will help you to address both of those issues as part of your recovery process. It should also be clear that this book contains a tool box of techniques and that you will be able to choose which ones best apply to your situation. This first part of this chapter consisted of Pain Reprocessing Therapy techniques that most people will need to incorporate into their recovery journey. Here we will introduce another major component of recovery: expressive writing exercises. In the following chapters, we will introduce Emotional Awareness and Expression Therapy (EAET) as well as several other concepts and techniques. Most likely, you will want to try many of these recovery tools, but you will not need to do ALL of them. Of course, the same is true for this section on expressive writing. I'd suggest trying at least some of the writing techniques that are presented here and also in the next few chapters. For some people, they are a key that leads to large changes in understanding yourself and in recovering from MBS. For others, they are helpful, but not essential and for still others, they play only a very small role, if any, in their recovery. Even though stressful life events may have triggered MBS, many people recover simply by using the PRT techniques described earlier in this chapter (and there will be other PRT techniques offered in the next couple of chapters). For some people, stressful life events are not a major cause of MBS, but rather it is learned neural circuits that were developed after an injury or an illness, such as a car accident or a viral infection. You can investigate your own situation and decide how to use this book. If you need help in figuring this out and in recovering, there are ample resources available to you by in person or remote access to online programs and individual or group coaching and therapy. See the appendix for some of these resources.

Many of the writing exercises in this program are based on insights from the therapeutic journaling movement and specifically on the excellent research of James Pennebaker (1990 and 2004). Dr. Pennebaker has shown that writing about stressful situations allows people to become healthier, develop perspective, and learn to let go of the reactions that have imprisoned them. He has also developed some specific writing activities that help do that, some of which we have incorporated into this program. We call them the Write Away Process, because you will be writing away your pain, anxiety, depression, and other symptoms.

The first week's writing exercise is called the 25-Minute Jog. I suggest that you try this process a few times and see how it feels to you. Many people have found it helpful to write about some of their stressful situations in order to uncover and express feelings that have been held inside, to release those feelings, to gain perspective on situations that may not have been apparent, and to move past those situations by being more caring and compassionate to yourself and often to others. This process can free you from some of the bonds that may have been a weight holding you back from living the life that best suits you.

Getting Started With the Write Away Process

Review the lists you made in the section, Addressing Stressors and Personality Traits on pages 116-117, of current and past stressors and personality traits you have compiled. Without spending too much time deciding, list the two to three items in each of the areas that you think are most likely influencing your health. You will be writing on these issues this week and probably for several weeks. You can write on one issue for several days if necessary, or you can write on a different issue each day. Use your intuition to decide what issues are most important and to decide when you can move on to write about other issues. Not everyone will need to do the writing exercises. You may have already processed the issues in your life or you may not find writing all that helpful. I'd suggest doing at least a few of these exercises initially and then decide how many you want or need to do. Do not think that you won't recover if you don't do each and every exercise in this book! Pick and choose those that fit you best.

When doing these exercises, you can choose between writing by hand, typing into a phone, tablet or computer, dictating or simply speaking out loud. Some people find that writing by hand is best, but of course some people have hand or arm pain that limits how much they can write, at least until they recover from MBS!

Current Stressors

1.
2.
3.

Past Stressors

1.

2.

3.

Personality Traits

1.

2.

3.

You will be learning two techniques for the first week's assignments: clustering and free-writing.

Clustering, also referred to as "webbing," is an effective way to brainstorm your way to self-discovery. Clustering allows you to access ideas quickly, using the circling of your ideas on paper to help you more easily go between the right and left hemispheres of your brain, an ability that's key to solving problems (Rico, 1983).

The five steps to producing a cluster are:

1. Choose one topic/issue from one of your lists (past stressor, current stressor, or personality trait). Write it in the center of the oval (next page). This is the nucleus of your cluster.

2. Set a timer for five minutes.

3. Begin to "free associate" on the topic/issue. Open your mind and write down whatever thought occurs to you. Write it down in a one- to four-word phrase, and then circle what you've written and connect it by a line to the nucleus.

4. Now you have two possibilities to prompt your thinking: what you wrote in your nucleus or what you just wrote in the satellite circle and connected to it. Now write down a word or phrase that represents your next immediate idea, circle it, and connect it to the circle that prompted it.

5. Continue this process until the timer signals your five minutes is up. You will end up with a cluster of ideas and thoughts, which may look like a web filling the page

Free-writing—or "fast writing" as it more appropriately might be called—is a powerful technique that allows you to access important pieces of information and understand them better. It is a way to gain perspective, which may serve to free you from some of the issues that have caused you pain and suffering. The idea behind it is that when you write faster than you normally would, helpful material that you would usually censor before even writing it down is allowed to surface.

Natalie Goldberg (1986) refers to the outcome of free-writing as "first thoughts," and among her six-step process, includes:

1. Keep your hand moving. Write faster than you would normally write in a reflective mood; attempt instead to take dictation from your thoughts as they stream across the radar screen of your mind.

2. Don't cross out anything, even if you didn't mean to write what you did.

3. Don't worry about spelling, punctuation, or grammar.

4. Write whatever comes into your mind or comes from your hand.

5. Allow any thoughts and any feelings to be expressed.

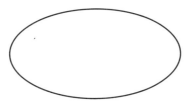

Beginning on this page, write the topic/issue from the nucleus of your cluster in the blank space of the sentence below.

Set a timer for ten minutes. Do free-writing on whatever thoughts the sentence sparks until your time is up. When writing, allow yourself to express any emotions that you might have. Express things as strongly as you wish. Use phrases such as "I feel ____" and "I felt _____" often.

Here are a few more tips about expressive writing. Do not make pain, anxiety, or depression the primary focus of your writing. That can reinforce those symptoms. Don't express resentment, anger, guilt, or shame towards yourself. These can lead to increased pain, anxiety, and depression. Instead, direct resentments or anger towards someone or some entity that you feel upset at. It is completely normal to have thoughts that are seen as negative, such as vengeful or jealous thoughts or wishing bad things towards others. When you are writing about negative thoughts or feelings, consider writing it on separate paper and destroying it when you are done. This symbolizes separating from these thoughts and feelings and letting them go. As you destroy the paper, tell yourself that you are not going to hang onto negative thoughts and emotions forever. You are going to let them go and move forward with your life.

My *feelings* about me and _____ include:

Set your timer for another ten minutes. The idea in the next exercise is to process your feelings. Expressing emotions is important, but it is also critical to understand them, gain perspective on them, and begin to move past them. Therefore, in this free-write, make sure to use phrases such as "I see that…," "I realize…," "I hope that…," "I need to…," "I want to…," "I can…," "I will…," "I understand that…," "I appreciate…," "I wonder if…," "I have learned…," and "I have discovered." Write whatever comes to your mind with a focus on understanding the topic/issue as best you can at this point in time. Of course, some feelings are likely to continue to be expressed, which is perfectly acceptable. The point of this section is to gain perspective on this situation or event so that you can move past it and allow it to stop bothering you. You may need to write about this particular issue a couple of times, but you can learn to let it go. There are three components of this process: being compassionate towards yourself and possibly others, letting go of the issue in your mind, and learning lessons from the situation in order to take actions to protect yourself as you move forward in your life. Therefore you can write about love for self and others as appropriate as well as about letting go of those for whom you will set boundaries for and/or choose to avoid as necessary. You can write about what you've learned from this issue and what actions you will take to protect yourself, be assertive regarding your needs, and connect to those you choose to love and befriend.

My *understandings* about me and _____ include:

You have just completed a 25-Minute Jog. It is common to feel relieved and in less pain after doing this writing exercise, but it is also not unusual to feel worse or have more pain. You are doing important work that deals with critical issues in your life, which have affected your mind and your body by causing MBS. Doing this work will free you from the symptoms of MBS, but it may not happen immediately. Sometimes people taking this program initially feel worse because they begin to stir up issues and emotions that were buried for a long time. They also might stir up conscious emotions or topics that they were unaware were affecting them so much. This is normal. Don't worry. In fact, if your symptoms either improve or worsen by doing the writing, that shows that these symptoms are truly caused by MBS. And when you see these symptoms change in any way (better, worse, moving from one spot to another, or shifting from one symptom to a different one), you are making progress!

In general, if your symptoms increase with these exercises, it is an indication that you have not fully resolved the issue and that it is still weighing on your mind. When you fully express your emotions (i.e., anger, guilt, sadness, and love, or letting go), you will usually feel much better right away. If you don't feel better, I'd suggest that you need to do more work on this issue. If you need help with this, find a trusted friend or therapist. Whatever you do, don't give up. Keep writing and keep doing this work. You will see changes within days or weeks.

For the rest of week one, do a 25-Minute Jog as you find useful. This may be doing one each day, or only a few times as necessary. You may decide to write about the same issue for several days or even all week, or you might decide you have finished with one issue and are ready to move to another one. You might find one issue too difficult to write on at first, and that's perfectly fine. You can approach it later as the program continues.

On the following pages, complete your 25-Minute Jogs for the first week. If you are unable to write on a certain day, don't worry. Do the best that you can. Remember not to be too hard on yourself. Do not beat yourself up. If you notice that you tend to be hard on yourself, you might want to do a 25-Minute Jog on that issue. Then you can practice being kind to yourself while you write.

Week One, Day Two:

Select a topic for today's free-write. Complete a five-minute cluster on this page. Then complete two ten-minute free-writes on the following pages.

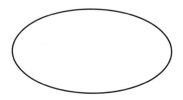

My *feelings* about me and _____ include:

My *understandings* about me and _____ include:

Week One, Day Three:

Select a topic for today's free-write. Complete a five-minute cluster for this page. Then complete two ten-minute free-writes on the following pages.

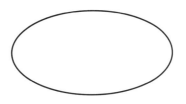

My *feelings* about me and _____ include:

My *understandings* about me and _____ include:

Week One, Day Four:

Select a topic for today's free-write. Complete a five-minute cluster for this page. Then complete two ten-minute free-writes on the following pages.

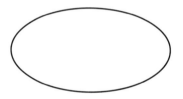

My *feelings* about me and _____ include:

My *understandings* about me and _____ include:

Week One, Day Five:

Select a topic for today's free-write. Complete a five-minute cluster for this page. Then complete two ten-minute free-writes on the following pages.

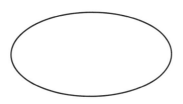

My *feelings* about me and _____ include:

My *understandings* about me and _____ include:

Week One, Day Six:

Select a topic for today's free-write. Complete a five-minute cluster for this page. Then complete two ten-minute free-writes on the following pages.

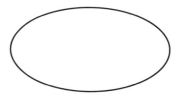

My *feelings* about me and _____ include:

My *understandings* about me and _____ include:

Week One, Day Seven:

Select a topic for today's free-write. Complete a five-minute cluster for this page. Then complete two ten-minute free-writes on the following pages.

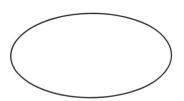

My *feelings* about me and _____ include:

My *understandings* about me and _____ include:

Reflections to Calm the Inner Mind

There are several reflective or meditative techniques that can be helpful in curing MBS and associated mind-body symptoms. You will learn them as you practice them. It is important to practice them in order to obtain the most benefit. The techniques you learn will last for your lifetime.

Meditation for Week One: Mindfulness Meditation

The first week's reflection is based upon the foundation of mindfulness meditation. I have been a mindfulness meditation teacher for over twenty years, and I have found it to be very helpful in learning to live life more fully, to appreciate what we have and who we are as a person, and to let go of things that have been or are bothering us. It is beyond the scope of this book to offer a comprehensive description of the philosophy and psychology of mindfulness meditation, which has existed for more than 2,500 years. Studies have shown that mindfulness can be effective in reducing pain and improving well-being (Kabat-Zinn, 1982; Grossman, et. al., 2007).

The basic concept of mindfulness is to learn to be focused, awake, and fully alive in the present moment. Mindfulness teaches us to face the present moment with interest and without judgment in order to be able to accept what has happened and learn that we cannot change what has happened. Once we accept the circumstances of the moment, we can make a good decision. We can decide to let go and move ahead to the next moment, to accept or to alter our reactions (thoughts and emotions) to what has occurred, or to act to change our situation. The philosophy of mindfulness teaches us that everything is transient and changing—our mood, our thoughts, our relationships, our family, our financial or work situation. It helps us understand that stress and pain are inevitable at different points in life. By practicing mindfulness, we learn that pain can be tolerated once we understand that we can control our response to it. For people with MBS, mindfulness can help to accept the past and to learn to choose our reactions to the present situation. Mindfulness teaches us to recognize and feel inner thoughts and emotions, to accept that they are there and that they will not harm us, and to let go of our reaction to them so that they don't continue to cause pain by keeping us locked into the stress and pain that emanates from our past.

You can listen to the Week One Meditation: Mindfulness Meditation, on a regular basis, or as often as it seems to be helpful. It will teach you techniques that you can use during the day as well.

You will find this meditation at unlearnyourpain.com, click on the Meditations tab at the top of the page and use this password: meditations. If you have trouble falling asleep, listen to it at night and it will help you fall asleep. Many people listen to it early in the morning, and this often helps them set the tone for their day. You can also listen to it when you are in pain to help you relax, cope better with the pain, and realize that you can learn to alter your focus to areas of your body that are not in pain, thus helping you be more in control of your pain. You can download the meditation to an MP3 player and listen to it while you are walking or during a break at work. However, I don't recommend listening to the meditation while driving—sometimes people fall asleep to it!

Meditation Synopsis

Find a place where you won't be disturbed. Begin this exercise by paying attention to your breath. You don't need to breathe in any particular pattern or depth, just notice your breath with interest and curiosity. Try not to judge your breath at all, just notice it as if you were noticing a fine painting. After some time, you will likely notice that your mind has wandered away from the breath, and when that happens, notice that the mind wandered and gently turn your attention to the breath. The essence of this practice is being able to notice what is on your mind and choosing to pay attention to that without reacting to it, and then choosing to pay attention to something else—for example, noticing the next breath.

Then begin to slowly scan through the body. Notice each and every body part with the same interested, yet non-reacting mind. When you arrive at parts of the body that are uncomfortable, notice the discomfort with less judging or reacting, accepting that things are the way they are for now, then choosing to move on to the next part of the body, paying attention in the same way. Do this exercise with kindness to the body. After scanning each part of the body, say to yourself, "I fully and completely accept myself and my body."

Take some time to notice your thoughts and feelings. Do this in the same way: noticing without reacting, accepting each thought or feeling as "just a thought" or "just a feeling," and letting go of each in order to notice the next one. In this way, you will be developing the ability to not be controlled by thoughts or feelings, but to choose which ones you pay attention to and which ones you just let go of. This will be important in breaking some of the associations that have developed between your thoughts and feelings and your MBS symptoms.

When emotions arise, allow your mind to notice how these emotions are connected to past traumas, to current stressors, to your personality, or to reactions that occur in either the child-mind or the parent-mind. Notice these mental phenomena without having to react to them. Notice the connection, accept that is the way your mind works, and choose not to react to it, choose not to allow those mental images to affect you, and just simply let them go, just as you let each breath go. At the end of this exercise, repeat to yourself three times, "I fully and completely accept myself and my body."

Using Mindfulness During Your Day

You can also use these techniques throughout the day. Simply by taking a few moments to focus on your breathing, you can train yourself to let go of something that may be annoying, upsetting, or worrisome. If you pay close attention to the breath for a few moments, you are letting go of everything else. You may be able to teach yourself to notice your breath when pain occurs, as a way of turning attention away from the pain.

When you can notice your thoughts with the awareness that they are "just thoughts" and that you don't have to be bothered by them, you don't have to act on them, and that you can just choose to let them go, you are taking a tremendous step towards freeing yourself from some of the chains that have imprisoned you into MBS. When you can do the same thing with emotions, such as fear, anger, guilt, shame, or worry, then you are closer to freeing yourself from the grip of pain that has been created by keeping these emotions inside of you.

From mindfulness practice, you learn that your body is strong and healthy. You can pay attention to all aspects of your body, not just the areas that hurt, and view your whole body as being well. The pain you experience due to MBS is transient. It will go away. You are learning not to worry about it, because you know what causes it. This is a critical point. Many people have used mindfulness to reduce pain without achieving much relief. This occurs when the cause of the pain has not been clearly diagnosed as being due to MBS (or when they have an ongoing structural cause for pain). When you know you have MBS, then you can see that the pain is being generated in your brain, just as are your thoughts. You can put the pain and your thoughts in the same category, as "just thoughts" and "just pain," nothing more; nothing to fear or worry about. You can co-exist with the pain or anxiety or depression and learn to separate yourself from it. This reduces fear, which allows the brain and the body to settle and reduce your MBS symptoms. Listen to this meditation, and practice living mindfully. It will not only help to free yourself from MBS, it will teach you to appreciate your life on a deep level.

chapter 8

Week Two: Finding Inner Strength

May I have the courage today
To live the life I would love,
To postpone my dream no longer,
But do at last what I came here for
And waste my heart on fear no more.
— John O'Donohue

It matters not how strait the gate,
How charged with punishments the scroll.
I am the master of my fate:
I am the captain of my soul.
— William Ernest Henley

Once you start doing this work, MBS symptoms often change. Sometimes, they start to get better and then get worse, or get worse for a short time before they get better. MBS symptoms can move from one part of the body to another or shift from one symptom, such as pain, to another one, such as fatigue, anxiety, or dizziness. These changes are all signs that you are able to alter the symptoms by changing your view of your symptoms and your reactions to them, which confirms that, and confirm that you are on the right track. Remember that you will be successful if you keep doing this work. The exercises in this program are relatively simple, but they are not always easy. It is hard work to face your own mind and body, which has been perpetuating your symptoms. But it is the work you must do to rid yourself of these symptoms and to improve your life.

After doing all of this preliminary work to calm the danger signal, most people will begin to see some changes in their symptoms. But even if you haven't seen any changes yet, don't worry! It can take several weeks or months to rewire the brain. So, please do not become discouraged or worried or upset. You will get there! Putting a timetable on your recovery tends to put more pressure on you and creates more fear and worry; not what you need right now.

Reprogramming the Brain: Pain Reprocessing Therapy, Advanced Techniques

The basic concepts of PRT are to interrupt the cycle of MBS symptoms leading to fear (and the rest of the other six Fs), leading to more symptoms over time. We accomplish this by completely changing your relationship to the symptoms, no matter what they are and no matter how severe they are. This requires a great deal of courage, but you can do it. The techniques presented in this chapter are an extension of the ones from chapter 7. They ask you to reverse as much fear, focus, fighting, frustration, trying to figure out and trying to fix your symptoms as you can. As you do this, you will be calming the danger signal in your brain to reduce and eliminate pain, anxiety, depression, fatigue, insomnia and any other MBS symptom you have.

Considering Symptoms as an Opportunity

Here I will be asking you to do something that is the opposite of your normal or typical reaction to the symptoms. You are aware that the usual reaction to symptoms is to avoid them and dread that they are coming. But these reactions indicate that you are afraid of the symptoms. Unfortunately, this fear tends to make them worse. So, here is a technique that you can use to reverse this. Instead of dreading the symptoms, you can try to look at them as opportunities. One of the best ways to reverse MBS is to meet the symptoms with calm and a smile! Therefore, it is better to actually look forward to the times when symptoms occur in order to have the opportunity to retrain your brain by using these processes we are describing here.

Sometimes, people get worried about this approach. Why would you want your symptoms to occur? You want to get rid of them, right? Of course, you do. However, the best way to get rid of them is to stop fearing them and one of the best ways to stop fearing them is to hope that they occur so that you get more opportunities to practice retraining your brain out of the pain neural circuits. When you can do that, you will be taking another huge step towards your recovery!

You can practice this simply by telling yourself and your brain that you hope that you get some of your symptoms today when you wake up in the morning; or when you go to work; or when you go about your day. You will tell your brain that you will meet all of these symptoms with a smile, knowing that you will be training the danger signal out of these symptoms by reminding your brain that these symptoms are not dangerous, they can't hurt you, and that they will be getting better over time.

Leaning into the Sensations

Here is another advanced technique that can be very helpful in reversing MBS. Once again, it is counter-intuitive. It goes against our natural impulse of trying to avoid the symptoms. Here, we are asking you to actually "lean in" to the sensation, which means to try to allow them to be there without fighting them, to allow yourself to tolerate them without fear, and to view them with curiosity and interest.

We all know that certain tastes that we can love are initially distasteful, such as dark chocolate, lemons, coffee, or beer and the same is often true for certain sensations, such as a deep massage or a hot sauna. At first taste, they are not pleasant, but with persistence, many people learn to enjoy them. Here, I am asking you to try to interpret the sensations of MBS differently. Rather than viewing them as uncomfortable, you are trying to make them less unpleasant. This may be difficult at times, of course, but with practice it is often possible to "lean in" to them, rather than running from them. Some people have found that they can "play" with the sensations, by watching how they shift or move or by putting an imaginary color on them or even some glitter. Give a different name to these sensations. You might call them "energy" or "warmth" or "tingling." It is just your brain generating weird or funny sensations that won't harm you, so you can learn to make them less unpleasant and even try to appreciate them in some way. For example, people with ringing in the ear (tinnitus) can begin to listen to the sounds as if they are a form of music, in order to reduce fear and focus. These are ways to change your relationship to the symptoms and train your brain that they are not dangerous. Try it little by little over time. This can make a huge difference.

Paradoxical Intention

Here is another method for lowering the danger signal. It is based upon the concept of paradoxical intention. Viktor Frankl wrote about this in his powerful book, *Man's Search for Meaning*, after World War II. He noted that the harder one tries to fall asleep, the more one doesn't fall asleep. And, he also noted, that if one tries to stay awake, they often fall asleep. This is one of the ways that our brains work: our brain does the opposite of what we are asking it to do. Telling the brain to turn off the pain may make things worse for some people. Yelling at the brain can fall into the same category. We don't want to be "at war" with ourselves.

So, you can use this form of "reverse psychology." If you tell a child: "Don't touch that, it's hot," the first thing they might do is touch it. Our subconscious brain is kind of like that.

Another concept that is useful here is the bully analogy. Bullies on a schoolyard playground will pick on other kids and say: "You're ugly" or "You're stupid." Then the kid will run or cry, and the bullies feed on that fear and do it more. But, the best way to stop a bully is to say back: "Those are good ones. Want to call me something else? Go ahead. I'm not afraid." This is a powerful response as it shows that there is no fear. It stops a bully who was feeding on the fear of his or her victim.

We know that fear of the mind-body symptoms is one of the main reasons for persistent symptoms. We want to stop the fear and using paradoxical intention is one very powerful way of showing no fear.

I sometimes call this technique, the Pat Benatar technique, as her song, Hit Me With Your Best Shot, describes this approach very well. "Hit me with your best shot, fire away…" is a message that you can start to give to your brain. You can only do this when you know that the pain or other symptom can't hurt you; you know that you're not damaged; and you know that you will recover. So, it doesn't matter if there is more pain for a while. It will go away. It will be temporary.

It's easy to practice this technique if you have the courage to do it. Empower yourself and be brave. When you get pain or another symptom, simply tell your brain to "Bring it on" or "Give me more" or "Make my day." Be serious and let the brain know that you're not kidding and that you're not afraid. Remember you are not yelling at your brain. You are just smiling and being fearless. See what happens as you do this. Most of the time, the brain will follow paradoxical intention and lower the pain, rather than raising it. If the pain does go up, that's fine. No matter, that also shows that it's the brain doing this. Just as a child having a temper tantrum, the tantrum may initially get worse before it gets better, but you just have to be patient and wait. You can again smile, knowing that you are not damaged or broken, and let the pain be there. It can't hurt you or harm you. And, as you keep giving your brain the message that you can handle it, you can take it, you're not afraid and simply "bring it," your brain will respond to your strength and power and it will turn the pain down! You'll see. Trust in this work.

Positive Affect

Another way to lower the danger signal is to create a positive mood. Many people with chronic pain or other symptoms find that they tend to become sad, depressed, angry and even hopeless over time. Unfortunately, these states of mind tend to make everything worse! Of course, it's hard to be happy when one is suffering with chronic pain or other debilitating symptoms. Yet, I have found that when people can move towards happiness, laughter, joy, grace, gratitude and awe, they feel better and their symptoms improve.

Here are some suggestions for ways to create a more positive mood. The first thing is to understand on a deep level that you are not broken, you are not damaged--either physically OR mentally! It can be a great relief to really know this, so please take some time to remind yourself of these facts: That you are healthy and that you are going to get better. Do this every day and make sure that you not only understand this, but also that you believe it. If you are having difficulty believing this, review the evidence sheet you created in chapter 5 or seek some guidance from some of the resources I recommend.

Second, we suggest that you take time to be grateful for as much as you can be grateful for in your life. You can do this by writing down a few things you are grateful for each day or by simply taking time to remind yourself of these things. Choose things that are both large, such as being alive, having a roof over your head, or having good relationships with some family and friends, AND for things that are small, such as a sunny day or a rainy day, flowers that are blooming or leaves that are changing, a nice interaction with someone in a store or someone letting you change lanes in traffic, or an order or delivery that worked well.

Third, you can find ways to laugh. Laughter is a powerful way to change the neural circuits in the brain. When you laugh, you are lowering the danger signal in the brain and you are even changing the expression of certain genes. The louder the laughter, and the longer the laughter, the more you are helping your brain to calm and feel safe. There are even societies devoted to getting people together just to laugh! Find things to do that are fun and enjoyable, especially if they are simple, such as playing card games or board games, learning how to do things that are silly, such as using a hula hoop, juggling, or other things. Look for ways to enjoy simple interactions, such as those with people who you meet in a restaurant, the post office, the grocery store, or anywhere. Take the time to talk to people about simple things, such as the weather, about how they think about their job, or any local activities. Spend time with people who you enjoy. Seek out phone or zoom calls with those who you are uplifting and understanding.

Fourth, find ways to just be happier. It may seem odd to say this, but you always have the opportunity to be happier and less depressed. It is often easy to focus on the things that are going wrong and the things that are bothering you. It often feels that so many things are overwhelming that it's impossible to be happy. And yet, you always have a choice. You can always choose how you respond to things that have occurred. You have the capacity to look on the bright side and have hope. You can choose happiness in any moment, even right now. You can take a deep breath and choose to smile and think about things that are hopeful and positive, even if there are many things that are the opposite. It feels good to choose happiness. You can take deep slow breaths and allow feelings of happiness to spread throughout your brain and your body. Try it!

And finally, you may have ways of connecting to spirituality in your life. There are many ways to be spiritual, which of course can include religious teachings and beliefs, but may also take the form of looking at the bigger questions of why we are here, what is our purpose, and what are the most important things in life. There is a sensation of awe that occurs when we focus on things that are much bigger than ourselves. Awe occurs when one prays, when one puts their faith in a higher power, when one sees a picture of the earth from space, when one sees a baby sleep or a toddler laugh, and when one contemplates the love and connection they feel with someone they trust. Consider taking time to participate in activities that create a sense of awe. You will know it when you feel it!

Thoughts

Everyone has loads of thoughts and feelings throughout the day. Surprisingly, most of these thoughts and feelings are actually subconscious; we are not aware of having them. But of course, we are aware of many thoughts and feelings, often so much so that we feel overwhelmed by them. After all you've learned about how the brain and the danger signal works, you probably won't be surprised to learn that it is the brain that creates all of our thoughts and feelings. And there are many! If you pay attention to these, you will see that you are literally bombarded with a whole variety of thoughts and feelings throughout the day. The thoughts are literally "all over the place:" thoughts about how your body feels right now, what you will have for dinner tonight, how your kids are, a work deadline or issue, the weather, a memory of your childhood, a song from the 90s, a commercial for an insurance company, and so much more. As you pay attention to your thoughts during the day, you will note that you may also have thoughts that are weird, silly, petty, and even evil. All of these are normal. Everyone has them. Most of these thoughts are meaningless and harmless and they just pass by without you barely noticing them. On the other hand, some of them may actually create a physical reaction of MBS.

One day I was walking into the kitchen, and I suddenly noticed a sharp pain that occurred in four spots in my back simultaneously. The pain lasted a few minutes and seemed to come from "out of the blue." I immediately stopped what I was doing and tried to notice what was going on in my mind. I asked myself, "What were you thinking about?" My first reaction was that I wasn't thinking about anything. So I asked again. This time it came to me. I'd been thinking about a conflict I was having with a relative.

Most people with chronic pain have many thoughts that I put into the category of "scary thoughts." We know that the danger signal in the brain can generate troublesome thoughts in the same way that it creates pain and other MBS symptoms. Many people with MBS have anxiety, depression, OCD and other syndromes that consist of scary and repetitive thoughts that can be overwhelming at times. It is critical to understand that this is simply another manifestation of MBS and that you can use the same techniques in this book for them as well. The danger signal will often activate more scary thoughts when it "sees" that you are not as fearful of the pain and other physical symptoms; or as those begin to lessen. The brain is still trying to "alert" you (or scare you), so it gives you different things to worry about. Don't be surprised at this. It's actually part of the recovery process. Another common reaction the danger signal has is to generate new and different physical symptoms or even symptoms that you had in the past, such as pain in an injury that healed years ago and hasn't bothered you for a long time.

Here are some common scary thoughts that most people with MBS have:

"Are we sure it's MBS/neural circuit issues? Another doctor told me that I had inflammation."

"The pain is so bad, it must be physical damage or an injury."

"I just can't believe that my brain is powerful enough to cause all of these symptoms."

"My body is tender or it seems twisted. Can that be caused by my brain?"

"I can feel the knots in my muscles and I have trigger points that need massaging so it must
be physical right?"

"I had a traumatic injury to the area which makes it hard to believe there's no damage."

"Even if this is MBS, can I really recover from all of this pain or after so many years?"

"How long will this take? I can't stand it anymore."

"I'm sure I will be the one who won't be able to do this."

I repeat: These are normal concerns and questions and you can realize that these worries
are also coming from the brain. They are part of MBS. They are just different manifestations of the
danger signal, trying to "alarm or alert" you; or simply trying to scare you. Don't be fooled! These are
just thoughts; nothing more. They are not reality. When I drive over a bridge, I often get the thought
that maybe I should turn the wheel hard to the right and flip the car over the railing. That's a scary
thought. If I take that thought seriously, I could fall into a deep hole of wondering why I have that
thought, why am I so depressed and suicidal, and how quickly can I find a therapist to help me. But
I don't do that. I step back from that thought and recognize that I'm not actually that depressed or
suicidal, but my brain gets that thought and it's not reality. (Of course, many people do have
depression or suicidal thoughts that do need addressing with therapy. If that is your situation, there
is no shame in seeking help while you work through this program.)

You can use the same process with these thoughts that you used in the during the day
exercise presented earlier in this chapter:

You can smile, take a nice slow breath, and say to yourself:

"That's interesting. That's my brain. This is just a thought. It's not important and can't harm
me. It will pass. I'm OK." Then take another slow breath and move on with your day.

The danger signal is like an over protective parent and it is trying to help you, protect you,
or alert you to danger. However, that danger is either no longer present or it is something you can
deal with.

Emotions

In addition to thoughts, you will see that you have loads of emotions that arise during each
day. Just as your thoughts are normal (even the ones that are scary or seem dangerous), your
emotions are normal as well. There are no bad or dangerous emotions. It is normal to feel strong fear

when life is filled with scary situations or to feel powerful anger when you have been hurt, attacked or betrayed. It is normal to feel deep sadness due to significant losses. These emotions have a purpose and are not in themselves dangerous. You can learn to identify these feelings when they arise and meet them without fearing them. You do not want to ignore them or suppress them or try to make them go away. You can allow yourself to feel these feelings, even though they may be strong, without pushing them away and you can learn to tolerate them and sit with them and express them in safe and healthy ways. They cannot harm you.

As you learn to identify emotions that arise, such as fear, anxiety, anger, guilt, or sadness, pay attention to how these emotions manifest themselves in your body. When you notice MBS symptoms, see if there are specific emotions that you can identify. Pay attention to your physical sensations and then see if you can identify any emotions that are also present just under the surface within you. There are often deep emotions underlying pain, anxiety, depression and other MBS symptoms. Encourage feelings of anger, guilt or sadness to rise up within you. They may be powerful, but you have the capacity to tolerate them and express them in a safe and private way; if you do this, the MBS symptom will often be reduced or alleviated. See how the emotion is manifested in your body without reacting to it. Let some of the feelings and physical sensations release, as you breathe, and observe them. Know that you are not in any danger, that these emotions are normal and that the physical sensations are manifestations of these underlying emotions.

Many people with MBS live in a state of heightened tension, their fight or flight reaction activated, living as if they are constantly in danger, as if everyday events are extremely dangerous and threatening. Become aware of when this happens and how you react. Only then can you begin to reduce this tension. When you notice these feelings, name them by saying to yourself: "Tension is here. Anxiety or fear is here." Know that these are transient, and you won't have to live with them forever. Observe how it feels, see how it affects your body, and breathe deeply in order to separate from the tension. You can then choose to tell yourself that you will pay attention to it again later and that there is no danger or threat right now. You can choose to pay attention to something else—the sky, a tree, another person—as a way of letting go. Move your body, change your location, or focus on a different part of your body. You may notice the symptoms are reduced or gone. As you do this, you will learn to recognize links between MBS and a wide range of emotions and you will gradually get better at feeling emotions and letting them go, reducing fear and other MBS symptoms.

While thoughts and emotions often create pain, there are many times when we are unable to identify a particular thought, emotion or stressful life event that might be connected to a symptom. This situation occurs more often than not. It is important to know this. Most of the time, you will not be able to find a cause for the onset of pain on a day-to-day basis. Don't worry about that. If you try too hard to find each thought or emotion, it will often be futile and can be counterproductive. It is enough to know that your symptoms are due to MBS; that they are temporary and will pass; that you are not damaged or broken; that your brain has learned these symptoms and that you are in the process of overcoming them by reducing fear and worry about them; and that you will get better. You just need to practice the exercises in this section on a regular basis. Please do not worry if your pain or other symptoms doesn't get better right away. Neural circuits, like bad habits, take time to reprogram. As long as you are reducing fear about these symptoms, you will get better. This practice is like training a puppy. You have to be persistent, consistent, patient and kind.

Meditation for Week Two: Embracing Emotions

The following is a meditation recorded on unlearnyourpain.com. Click on the Meditation tab at the top of the page and put in the password: meditations. Select the Embracing Emotions meditation.

Try this exercise when you are feeling a symptom of MBS, such as pain, anxiety, depression, or fatigue. Close your eyes and experience the symptom without being distracted from it. Know that it can't harm you, but allow yourself to feel it in your mind or body, and notice how it may vary moment by moment. Feel it fully then see if you can feel what lies underneath it. Usually you will find worry and fear. Feel these feelings and let them grow without being distracted from them. See how they feel in your body and what parts of your body are reacting. After doing this, search underneath the fear for other emotions. See if you can feel any anger or resentment, and see how that feels in your body; also look for any guilt, and then move towards sadness and grief. Allow these feelings to blossom within you and see how you experience them. Let tears come as they will. Finally, search underneath these for feelings of compassion for yourself. Look for caring and kindness. Breathe deeply and sit with these feelings for awhile. Notice what happens with the MBS symptom that you started with; see if it has shifted; it will often disappear as the other emotions are felt.

Writing Exercise for Week Two: Unsent Letters

As you are now well aware, one of the causes of MBS is holding emotions inside. We often are unable to express some of these emotions verbally for a variety of reasons. The person we need to talk to may be gone from our lives, unavailable, or simply impossible to talk to. There are some things that one simply can't express to a boss, neighbor, or relative. Many emotions stem from many years ago, and the person involved may have changed. Yet we still may be hanging on to feelings that have been bothering us for years or decades. One way to express these feelings in a safe and useful way is to write letters that we do not send (Rainer, 1978).

Unsent letters are useful to express negative feelings that we have been harboring and that are causing us harm, such as unexpressed anger, resentment, fear, guilt, or shame. However, it is also important to express gratitude and thankfulness to those whom we may have not had a chance to thank. Sometimes, we need to write letters of love, apology, or regret to those who are now missing from our lives.

Create a list of possible recipients to whom you might send an unsent letter. These letters will allow you to explore whatever you need to explore regarding your relationships. You may need to write to a parent, relative, current or former spouse, significant other, child, friend, neighbor, colleague, boss, or coworker. You may need to write to someone who has died or a person from whom you are estranged, as well as to people who are present in your life today. You can write to groups of people or to a president, a Pope, or God. It is often useful to write a letter to different aspects of yourself. You can write letters to your pain, to your subconscious mind, or to different aspects of your personality. You can write a compassionate letter to your younger self or to your future self who is happier, more at peace, and free of pain, anxiety and depression. As mentioned before, you may not need to do any or all of these exercises. Try a few initially and see how you respond. Then complete as many as you want or need to do.

My list of possible "recipients" of an unsent letter includes:

_____

_____

_____

_____

_____

_____

_____

_____

_____

_____

_____

_____

Each day, you will be choosing one of the recipients listed to write an unsent letter to. Take a look at your list now, and circle the people that you think it might be most helpful for you to write to first. Once you begin writing, you may discover you need to send several letters to the same person. Feel free to do this if necessary. Then you may choose to move on to other letters.

When you write, feel free to allow your mind and hand to write whatever needs to be said to the person or entity you've chosen to address. Since the letter will not be sent, you can say anything that comes to your mind without censoring it. You might choose to use profanity, for example, or to express extreme emotion. This is perfectly acceptable and can help to relieve tension in the subconscious mind. Know that you can destroy any of these letters after you've written them. This is a way to leave them behind you and let go of the issues you've addressed. It also makes sure that no one else will be reading them.

Trust that you are safe in writing this letter and that you can express any thoughts or feelings that cross your mind. Write as long as you need to, but typically ten to fifteen minutes is reasonable. Use additional pages if you need more space. When you start writing, you may be surprised by the strength of the emotions you have been holding in.

After each letter, reflect on and write a description of what lessons you have learned from this person, what you have gained from your interaction with this person (even if the interaction was very destructive), and in what ways you may have grown as a result of your relationship with this person. State how you've been able to deal with any issues related to this relationship and what actions you will be taking going forward. Write these reflections in a letter to yourself. See Rainer (1978) for more information on this type of writing.

Week Two, Day One:

Date and write a letter below to a person or entity from your unsent letter list. Express your thoughts and feelings fully. Use as much paper as needed. Remember to sign your name.

Dear _____,

Write a letter to yourself reflecting on the unsent letter you just finished. What have you learned from this person or your interaction? What have you learned from writing this letter? How have you dealt with any issues related to this relationship? How do you plan on dealing with these issues in the future?

Dear _____,

Week Two, Day Two:

Choose a recipient for today's unsent letter.

Dear _____,

Write a letter to yourself to reflect upon the letter you just wrote.

Dear _____,

Week Two, Day Three:

Choose a recipient for today's unsent letter.

Dear _____,

Write a letter to yourself to reflect upon the letter you just wrote.

Dear _____,

Week Two, Day Four:

Choose a recipient for today's unsent letter.

Dear _____,

Write a letter to yourself to reflect upon the letter you just wrote.

Dear _____,

Week Two, Day Five:

Choose a recipient for today's unsent letter.

Dear _____,

Write a letter to yourself to reflect upon the letter you just wrote.

Dear _____,

Week Two, Day Six:

Choose a recipient for today's unsent letter.

Dear _____,

Write a letter to yourself to reflect upon the letter you just wrote.

Dear _____,

Week Two, Day Seven:

Choose a recipient for today's unsent letter.

Dear _____,

Write a letter to yourself to reflect upon the letter you just wrote.

Dear _____,

Rebuilding Your Life

In order to advance beyond the ruts that we tend to get stuck in, it may be necessary to rebuild some aspects of our lives. Sometimes people with chronic pain or other symptoms lose the ability to function in their usual ways or feel stuck in their lives. Consider these thoughts as you complete the exercises for this week.

1. Decide that you can be pain free (or symptom free).

It is possible for you to get better. Develop and maintain this attitude, and remind yourself of this daily. Since there is nothing permanently wrong with your body, you will be able to feel better as you work through this program. It may take some time, but do not give up hope. If you keep working on this program, you will understand yourself better and understand the relationship between the mind and the body. These understandings, along with practicing the exercises, will help you get better.

2. Figure out what you want to do.

Given that you are going to get better, you can consider your next steps. It is critical to have a purpose in life. Begin to ask yourself questions such as: What are my skills? What things do I really like to do? What work would bring me pleasure and be meaningful? How can I make my current job more meaningful and pleasurable? What leisure activities are meaningful and bring me pleasure? How can I contribute to the world, to my community, to the people around me, to my family? What things do I need to leave behind or let go of? What parts of myself do I need to let go of, and what parts of myself do I want to nourish or emphasize? Are there certain people who you need to spend more time or reconcile with? Are there some people who you need to set some boundaries with or distance yourself from?

3. Look at the big picture.

Take some time each day to think about life in general. Consider your gifts, what you have been given by others, and the material things you have. Be grateful for what you have. Consider the role of religion or spirituality in your life. Ask yourself what is important to you and what you might do in small ways on a regular basis to improve your life and the lives of others around you.

4. Possibility

Consider any and all possibilities for yourself. Picture a future that includes a healthier and a more productive you. Begin to include elements of that "new you" into your day, every day. When you wake up in the morning, envision some of these possibilities and carry them with you throughout the whole day.

5. Kindness to self

One of the most important aspects of ridding yourself of MBS and improving your psychological health is be kind to yourself. I cannot emphasize this enough. It is very easy to develop and maintain a self-critical attitude that can block recovery from MBS. I urge you to take time each day to be kind to yourself. You can do this by listening to meditations, by doing the writing exercises, by catching yourself in self-critical thoughts, and by doing some things for yourself. This is a simple yet powerful aspect of this program.

If you miss doing some of the homework, be kind to yourself. If you forget a task or don't finish all the work or errands on your list, be kind to yourself. Here are some examples of what I mean by being kind to yourself:

- Accepting that you are human and that you cannot be everything to everyone.
- Accepting your faults and realizing that you are a good person.
- Forgiving yourself for your mistakes, just as you would forgive others whom you love.
- Learning to say "no" to certain requests.
- Sending positive and caring messages to yourself.
- Recognizing that many others have been in your situation and have survived and thrived.
- Accepting your feelings as being normal.
- Catching yourself when you send critical messages to yourself and replacing those with kind and understanding messages.
- Figuring out what you need and not being shy about asking for it or taking steps to attain it.
- Taking time for yourself to do things just for you or just to allow you to relax and enjoy life.
- Standing up for yourself.
- Realizing that you are an important person on this earth and that you deserve to be happy and healthy.

Take some time for the following exercise, which was adapted from the excellent book, *The Mindful Path to Self-Compassion* by Christopher Germer.

Place your hand over your heart and breathe deeply. With each in-breath, inhale kindness and compassion for yourself. Allow kindness to fill you as it fills your lungs. Feel the warmth of compassion as it soothes you and calms you. Let that warmth spread to your whole body.

Notice any areas of your body that are tense or painful. Direct the kindness and compassion that you are generating to that part. Allow that body part to relax and let go of the tension. Direct kindness to all of your body.

Notice any negative emotions that are present. Direct compassion to these emotions. Accept them as normal reactions and allow them to pass as you direct kindness to them and to yourself.

Breathe out the tension from your body and mind. Let pain and negative emotions be released. Send them out and let them go.

Finally, send out kind thoughts and wishes to others in your life. Send kind thoughts and wishes to people in your neighborhood or city.

6. Develop a plan of action for the week.

What activities can you do this week that will further your recovery? Decide that you are going to do physical activities that are good for you, such as walking or exercising. Plan to do some mental activities that are good for you, such as reading a book, doing crossword puzzles, or playing cards or board games. Make sure that you do something pleasurable for yourself each week, such as seeing a movie, taking a hot bath, or getting a massage. Agree to see other people in comfortable surroundings, such as going to church or getting together with friends for coffee, a meal, or for a walk.

Most people with MBS tend to think more about others and do more things for others than they do for themselves. If you are one of these people, it is critical that you begin to take some time for yourself each week. Arrange your schedule to do this. Ask those around you to help you find this time. Do not let this time be taken away from you. Find activities that will be enjoyable and fun, and make sure that you do them without feeling any guilt about taking time for yourself. You need this time for your healing process.

When you consider which activites to do, think about the triggers which have become connected to your pain or other MBS symptoms. As you will recall, triggers are learned responses in your brain and need to be overcome for complete healing. The more you encounter these triggers and reprogram your brain to overcome them, the quicker you will get better. When you continually avoid the triggers, you give them more power over you. Plan to overcome some triggers this week.

On the following list, write down some things that you might like to do in the next week, the next month, and in the next six months to one year. Feel free to put down anything that appeals to you. You are not making a commitment to do any of these right now; you are brainstorming about ideas that would improve your life or give you happiness.

Exercise: Things I Would Like to Do

Activities that will be productive and/or overcome triggers:

This week:

In the next month:

In the next six months to one year:

Things that are just for me:

This week:

In the next month:

In the next six months to one year:

Things I can do for others that would give me pleasure:

This week:

In the next month:

In the next six months to one year:

During this week, pick out one or two things from each of the above categories and see if you can do them. Plan ahead, and make sure you can accomplish them. You are doing them for yourself, and you deserve to do them. You deserve to be happier and to be free of MBS symptoms. And it is important to realize that as you become happier in your life and more comfortable with yourself, you will be taking big steps towards unlearning your pain.

chapter 9

Week Three: Dialogues Towards Understanding

Our own life is the instrument with which we experiment with truth.
— Thich Nat Hanh

Working with Emotions: Healing the Inner Hurts

By now, it should be obvious that there are powerful links between emotions and symptoms such as pain, fatigue, insomnia, anxiety, and depression. The same areas of the brain are activated by both physical injuries and emotional injuries. Emotional memories are permanent and emotional hurts that occurred in the past do not necessarily disappear over time. When one looks very carefully at the life stories of people with MBS, the patterns that cause MBS are usually clear. Lessons learned early in life create pathways that are stored in the danger/alarm mechanism of the brain. If there are severe early life stressors, MBS symptoms may begin immediately and may persist for many years. Often early life stressors do not cause the development of symptoms at that time; however stressful events that occur later in life may trigger these stored emotional hurts causing MBS symptoms to develop. This is particularly common when the situation later in life is quite similar in an emotional sense to the earlier life situations, but may also occur with stress in general.

The emotions that are most commonly held in this emotional memory are fear, anger, guilt, shame and sadness or grief. Typically, individuals are most aware of their fear, as this represents the usual response to being hurt, especially by those who are closest to us. Holding onto fear eventually leads to the anxiety disorders of OCD, PTSD, social phobia, and panic disorders, which are manifestations of a runaway flight reaction. When we become overwhelmed with fear, the freeze or submit reaction can be activated with resulting depression and/or fatigue.

The second response to emotional injury is anger and resentment. Anger is a much healthier response to being hurt than is fear. When one is trapped and powerless, fear is manifest. However when one is powerful, it is possible to express anger and to overcome someone who is causing us harm. Anger is a manifestation of the innate fight reaction of the autonomic nervous system. It occurs when we protect ourselves by acting in an assertive manner. Most children who are hurt emotionally are powerless to express their anger and thus they learn to hold anger in. A life-long pattern of feeling afraid and the inability to express anger or assert oneself may develop and these are the basic building blocks for MBS. Learning to overcome that pattern of holding anger in, beginning to stand up for yourself and be more assertive are often components in unlearning your pain.

The other set of emotions that often promotes the development of MBS are guilt and shame. There are two forms of guilt, conscious guilt and subconscious guilt. Conscious guilt consists of the feelings that many people have for things that they regret having done. Many people with MBS tend to feel guilty for many things they have done and they have a difficult time letting go of that guilt or forgiving themselves, even though they will quickly forgive others for similar actions. Even if you do not experience conscious guilt, subconscious guilt is often present. There is one form of subconscious guilt that is important to recognize, i.e., the guilt one feels for the resentment and anger that is held towards others, particularly those closest to us such as our parents, siblings, spouses, and children. This type of guilt is common. Facing it can lead to release of grief and open the door to true healing. Finally, shame is a powerful blocker of healing. Shame is the belief that one isn't a good person, isn't worthy of being loved, or doesn't deserve to be happy. People who were not fully loved or accepted in their childhood or who were frequently told that they weren't good enough, or smart enough, or attractive enough tend to develop shame. Guilt and shame are forms of anger being turned inward upon oneself. They often must be consciously dealt with in order to reverse MBS.

Stressful situations either in childhood or later in life cause losses, such as the loss of the physical presence or affection from important people in our lives. It is only natural that these losses will cause sadness and grief. As with the other major emotions, sadness and grief often need to be experienced, expressed, and released in order to fully heal from Mind Body Syndrome.

Finally, the emotion that everyone longs to experience is love. When we are able to truly experience love, caring, and kindness towards ourselves and towards others, healing on a deep level occurs and MBS symptoms melt away. It is not difficult to see that holding onto anger and resentment towards others will block the ability to love them fully. It is also obvious that turning anger towards ourselves by holding onto guilt, being unable to forgive ourselves, and living with shame will block the ability to love oneself. Many people with MBS are unable to say that they are a good person or that they love themselves. The exercises in this book are designed to release suppressed anger, let go of guilt and shame, allow grief to be experienced, and then move towards loving relationships with oneself and the important people in our lives. When you do this, the old anxieties and fears do not weigh upon you and the normal stress of everyday life becomes more easily manageable. This path is surprisingly simple to accomplish, although it takes courage to recognize deep emotions that have long been held in and to allow ourselves to feel them and express them. However, it is well worth the effort as it is a path that is truly healing, both in mind and body.

Emotional Awareness and Expression Therapy

As mentioned earlier, Mark Lumley and I developed Emotional Awareness and Expression Therapy (EAET) as a way to guide people towards dealing with emotional hurts, both present and past. I have also explained that not everyone with MBS will need to engage in this type of emotional processing work. You can read these sections and decide if they make sense to you or apply to your situations. You can also try some of these exercises to determine if they will be useful to you. Or you can come back to them later, if you feel the need to do so.

We developed EAET as a relatively simple way of accessing powerful emotions that may have been held inside for some time. This process, as is the case for most therapies, was built upon the work of others. The therapy that we drew on most heavily was Intensive Short-Term Dynamic Psychotherapy (ISTDP). ISTPD was developed by Dr. Habib Davanloo, a psychiatrist from Montreal (Davanloo, 1978, 1990, 1999). He realized that the deeply buried emotions of anger, guilt, and grief were the sources of anxiety, depression, and chronic pain. He understood that we tend to cover up and suppress these emotions because they are uncomfortable, so we develop a variety of defenses (techniques for blocking anger and guilt). Dr. Davanloo discovered that uncovering and releasing these deeply held emotions were healing and often the healing occurs very rapidly once these emotions are mobilized. I learned about this type of therapy from Dr. Allan Abbass in Halifax, Nova Scotia. He has conducted several research studies that document the power of this therapeutic approach (Abbass, et. al., 2002, 2003, 2008, 2009, 2010). This model is also described succinctly by David Malan and Patricia Coughlin Della Selva in *Lives Transformed* (2006) and in the book by Dr. Abbass entitled *Reaching Through Resistance* (Abbass, 2015). If you want to access ISTDP in its original form, please see the above references. Dr. Abbass and I have combined on a book designed for clinicians describing our approach to MBS/psychophysiological disorders, entitled *Hidden From View.*

The following case studies illustrate how EAET can be used to address emotions that have occurred at any point in one's life. I will describe in detail how to use EAET for yourself later in this chapter. In these cases, you will get a sense of the process. These are dramatic examples. Your situation may be very different and the process you use may be as powerful as these cases or it might be done with much less of emotional output. Each situation is unique and requires differing levels of emotional expression.

Dealing with Anger

Michael is a thirty-eight-year-old man who suffered with severe migraine headaches. For the past ten years, he had had a headache every day despite seeing top headache specialists who treated him with more than fifteen different medications. When I met him, he wore dark glasses because bright light triggered headaches, he wore earplugs because loud sounds triggered headaches, and he couldn't go outside in inclement weather. He told me that his father was a "rage-oholic" and an alcoholic who caused Michael to have a childhood of abuse and humiliation. The headaches were triggered when his wife rejected him and filed for a divorce. In addition, she made it difficult for him to see his son thus preventing him from becoming the kind of supportive father he desperately wanted to be, rather than the type of father he himself had. He had completed the process described in chapter 5 and clearly understood that the headaches were caused by his emotional reactions to the way his father treated him and the stress of the divorce and his separation from his son.

I employed the EAET model with him and here is an approximate transcription of the conversation between us:

Dr. S.: Tell me about a time when your father was particularly abusive.

M: We were at a wedding, and I was about seven years old. I made a comment about liking someone's watch. It seemed pretty innocent to me. However, my father became enraged. He started yelling at me and he slapped me. Then he made me stand in the corner of the room for the rest of the wedding.

Dr. S.: How did that make you feel?

M: I felt hurt.

Dr. S.: So, you were hurt. That's it, only hurt? (voice rising)

M: Yes, I was hurt. There was nothing I could do.

Dr. S.: You were hurt. He hurt you, yes? You were powerless. There was nothing you could do. Were you angry with him?

M: Yes, I was angry.

Dr. S.: Are you still angry? Does it bother you that he treated you that way? (voice rising)

M: Yes, it bothers me.

Dr. S.: So, let's do something about it. You don't want to stay hurting your whole life, do you? You're hurting now, both physically and mentally, right? You have horrible pain. Do you want to keep that pain or let it go?

M: No, I am tired of it.

Dr. S.: Good. That makes sense. You can do that and you can start right now. So, let's be that child of seven. You've just been put in the corner, just been slapped, just been yelled at. You didn't do anything wrong. How do you feel inside?

M: Hurt.

Dr. S.: That's it. No anger?

M: Yes, I'm angry.

Dr. S.: You're whispering. Do you feel angry or not? (voice rising)

M: Yes, I'm angry. (louder now)

Dr. S.: OK. You're angry. Are you really angry or just pretend angry?

M: Yes, I'm really angry!

Dr. S.: OK, say it: Father, I'm angry at you!

M: Father, I'm angry at you!

Dr. S.: You have no right to hit me!

M: You have no right to hit me!

Dr. S.: My anger is justified!

M: My anger is justified!

Dr. S.: Again!

M: I'm angry, you have no right to hit me, my anger is justified. I don't deserve to be treated that way.

Dr. S.: No one does!

M: No one does!

Dr. S.: Do you feel this anger in your body?

M: Yes.

Dr. S.: Where do you feel it?

M: In the pit of my stomach.

Dr. S.: Yes, I see. It makes you sick. It's sickening what he did to you!

M: Yes, disgusting.

Dr. S.: Right. But you are holding back some, keeping the emotions in, inside your stomach area. Do you see that? There's a tendency to hold those feelings inside. And they are painful; they are pain. Why don't we work on getting them stronger, getting them up and out? Are you with me?

M: OK, yes, I'm with you.

Dr. S.: OK. Great. You're doing great. Let's start again. You're standing in the corner. You're a little boy, only seven. Hit, yelled at, humiliated. Can you feel that? Are you there? What does that child need to say, to express, to become powerful and free?

M: Yes, I feel it. The child says, "Father, I hate you. You have no right to do that to me. You've treated me this way too many times, for too long."

Dr. S.: Yes, again!

M: I'm angry. I'm mad. I won't stand for it. I deserve to be treated better!!

Dr. S.: And?

M: I'm pissed. This is wrong. I'm angry. Stop it! Stop it!

Dr. S.: Do you feel that anger in your body?

M: Yes.

Dr. S.: Where in your body?

M: In my throat, in my head, my hands.

Dr. S.: Good. What does the anger do? What does it do to your father to get him to see, to get him to stop? Not what you do, but what does that anger do, right now?

M: It yells at him. It tells him to stop.

Dr. S.: Good. It yells at him. Talks back, stands up for you.

M: Yes.

Dr. S.: Does he listen? No. He's not listening. The anger has to try harder. What does it do now?

M: It moves towards him. Leaves the corner.

Dr. S.: Yes, and then what does it do?

M: It pushes him, shoves him. (voice getting stronger)

Dr. S.: Yes, that what it needs to do. But he's still yelling. What does it do then?

M: It pushes him into a corner, corners him.

Dr. S.: Yes, that's right. Then what does it do? What does it have to do to really make him hear, to make him understand?

M: It hits him, kicks him. It kicks and kicks and kicks. (voice loud and strong)

Dr. S.: Again and again?

M: Yes, again and again.

Dr. S.: It doesn't stop. Is he still talking?

M: Yes, he's still talking, and the anger doesn't stop. It keeps on kicking, over and over. (voice firm and fierce)

Dr. S.: Until what happens.

M: Until he can't talk. He can't talk anymore. He's quiet.

Dr. S.: Is he bleeding? Is he unconscious?

M: Yes, he's bleeding some, he's passed out, unconscious. Just lying there. (voice softer now)

Pause…

Dr. S.: And how do you feel then?

M: I feel relaxed, relieved. (takes a deep breath)

Dr. S.: Do you feel bad about what the child did?

M: No.

Dr. S.: Yes, it needed to do that.

Pause…

Dr. S.: When you look at your father now, as a grown man, not as a child anymore, how do you feel towards him now?

M: I love him. I care about him. He had a problem. (a few tears in his eyes)

Dr. S.: Yes, he did. How do you feel now?

M: Sad, but also much better.

In this interaction, Michael was able to let go of the hurt and humiliation enough to become powerful and express the inner rage that had been held in his mind and body for so many years. He overcame the subconscious guilt about feeling anger towards his father. He allowed the anger to rise to the surface and allowed it to bubble over in a metaphoric way. He fully expressed the anger verbally in order to "vanquish" the father who had abused him. This powerful act released long-held suppressed anger and his body immediately relaxed. The anger is not the anger he currently has towards his father, but the anger that child had towards his father. Once it was expressed and cleared out, he could be free to express sadness and love towards his father in the present. He later told me of a dream he had where his father was a puppet held up by strings made of alcohol.

I asked him to do some therapeutic writing exercises that are described in this program. He wrote about understanding and having pity for his father. He wrote about having understanding and compassion for himself as a child. He clearly understood how the events in his life led to his headaches. His headaches lessened immediately. Over the course of a few days, he stopped wearing dark glasses and earplugs and he was able to sit outside when it was raining. He has only had the beginning of a few headaches since then. When the headache pain starts, he stops and reminds himself that he does not have a serious disease; he observes the pain and asks himself what event has just occurred, what he was thinking of, or if he is feeling some emotion. Usually there is an event or an emotion present that has caused his body to react. He is now able to recognize emotions such as resentment or anger, sadness, or guilt, and let them in, look at them, express them, act on them if necessary, and let them go. He is currently not taking any medication for migraine headaches and is able to spend quality time with his father.

Dealing with Anger Mixed with Guilt

Many people with Mind Body Syndrome have had emotionally traumatic experiences in their lives, often very early in their lives. When people are powerless to affect these situations, their anger is typically suppressed or expressed towards others later in life. People with traumatic experiences early in life often need to fully express these feelings by allowing the anger to well up and (metaphorically) overpower the offending person. They may not feel a great deal of guilt about their anger (as they feel so much better after the "child" has become powerful for the first time), as demonstrated in the case of Michael above. However, traumatic experiences that occur later in life can often be resolved without that metaphoric release, yet there may be a great deal of guilt associated with the situation. The case of Edward is a case in point.

Edward sought my help for back pain that had been present for several years. Medical testing had not demonstrated any significant structural disorder and traditional medical treatments didn't help. He works as an engineer and likes to have everything in order. He works at an auto company, is married, and has two children. His first child was a "perfect" daughter and everything was going well until his second daughter arrived. Over the years, this daughter had a great deal of problems, both emotionally and behaviorally. These issues were so upsetting to him that he began to show anger in many different settings. His back pain began during this time and didn't resolve even after his daughter moved out of the house and began to act more responsibly. Here is the session where he worked on these issues.

Dr. S.: So, when your daughter was a teenager, she was difficult.

Ed: Yes, unbelievable. She created tons of chaos; chaos in our family, chaos in my life.

Dr. S.: So, how did you feel about that?

Ed: It was horrible! It drove me crazy. I found myself punching walls in our home and I've never done anything like that before.

Dr. S.: So, you had a lot of anger?

Ed: Yes, tremendous anger and I didn't know how to handle it. It tore me up inside, tore up our family. Now I see that it was what caused my back to hurt, although I never realized that before.

Dr. S.: So, let's see if we can get some of this anger up and out. Are you willing to try?

Ed: OK, where do we start?

Dr. S.: Let's pretend that your daughter is sitting right here. You are in the midst of the worst times, not now, but then, when she was acting out, being disrespectful, using drugs, failing school. What were your feelings then?

Ed: I was upset, hurt, angry.

Dr. S.: So, you were angry. How angry?

Ed: I had a tremendous amount of anger.

Dr. S.: Pretend that she's right here. Tell her exactly how you felt, don't hold anything back.

Ed: I am so angry at you. You lie, you swear, you don't do anything to help. You're not even going to school. I can't stand it.

Dr. S.: Yes, you're angry. Go on. Let it all out.

Ed: I hate you. I hate you. You ruined our family. You've ruined my life. Everything was fine until you came along. (voice rising) And I'm pissed. Why did you do this? Don't you care about anyone else?

Dr. S.: Yes, more, more.

Ed: I can't do anything with you. I can't do anything for you. I'm so furious that I wish you were never born! (stops speaking, breathing quickly)

Dr. S.: I see. That must have been horrible. You were in a horrible spot. Nothing you could do; no way to solve the problem. No wonder you were punching walls.

Ed: Yes, I was trapped, powerless, and full of resentment and rage.

Dr. S.: That would be enough to cause back pain in anyone. You were so hurt, so angry, but couldn't really express the anger or do anything about it.

Ed: Yes, no doubt. I see that.

Dr. S.: Now, when you look back at that situation from where you are now, do you have any regrets? Are there any regrets about how you treated your daughter? Any regrets about anything you've said just now?

Ed: Yes. Yes, many.

Dr. S.: OK, now from the point of view of today, imagining your daughter sitting here once again. What do you want to say to her now?

Ed: I am so sorry. I didn't know what to do. I didn't know how to act, what to say. I wanted to help you, but I couldn't.

Dr. S.: Yes, you're sorry. How sorry?

Ed: I am so sorry. (begins to tear up) I love you. I didn't want to hurt you. I just wanted things to be right, to be good. I couldn't take it, and I took it out on you. I'm sorry. I love you. I wish I could do things differently. (crying)

Dr. S.: Yes, it hurts, doesn't it? This is what you need to say, too.

Ed: Yes, I need to say this. I need to tell her.

One week later, Ed's back pain was 90% better and he spent several hours with his daughter. He told me that this was the best time he's ever had with her. He felt so much better about himself and their relationship. For the first time, Ed had been able to discharge the anger that he carried towards his daughter (in a safe, therapeutic fashion), release the guilt that he'd been carrying for several years, and bring feelings of caring and compassion towards his daughter to the forefront of his mind.

Working with Anger, Guilt, Grief, and Love

A forty-five-year-old man by the name of Chris came to see me for anxiety. He had severe episodes of anxiety caused by work and life stress. He had no difficulties in childhood until the tragic sickness and death of his mother when he was sixteen years old. Following her death, his father was not able to comfort him or support him. His father immersed himself in his work and Chris was left to his deal with his feelings on his own. Chris spiraled into problems with school leading to detentions and eventually expulsion from his high school. Over the years, he had stabilized his life, gotten married and had children, but he continued to be plagued with anxiety.

I introduced the EAET model to help him understand how his deep feelings had been held inside and never expressed or processed. I explained that these feelings were the cause of his current difficulties and that he would have a much easier time in dealing with the anxiety once he dealt with these deep emotions. He affirmed that he was willing to do this work and we began.

> **Dr. S.:** So, tell me how you felt when your mom passed away.
>
> **C:** I was very hurt. I felt alone and sad.
>
> **Dr. S.:** Of course, that makes sense. How else could you feel?
>
> **C:** It was a hard time and I've worked hard to get past it.
>
> **Dr. S.:** Does it still hurt when you think about it? Right now, if you put yourself in that place, that place of the sixteen-year-old boy, does it still hurt?
>
> **C:** Yes, yes it does.
>
> **Dr. S.:** After your mom passed away, did you have any resentment at all? Any anger because she died?
>
> **C:** Yes, to some degree, but I'm not an angry person.

Dr. S.: Yes, of course, but were you angry at all that she died?

C: Yes, I was.

Dr. S.: If you put yourself into the shoes of that sixteen-year-old boy, does he have any anger? What does he say?

C: Why did this have to happen? It's not fair, it's not right!"

Dr. S.: Yes, what else does he say?

C: She shouldn't have died. I'm upset.

Dr. S.: Of course, express the anger that you felt.

C: I'm angry. It's not fair!

Dr. S.: Good. Who are you angry with?

C: I don't know, not my mom.

Dr. S.: So, are you angry with God? With whom?

C: I don't know, just angry.

Dr. S.: Is any of that anger towards your mom? I know it wasn't her fault. Of course, she didn't want to leave you. She loved you. But she did leave you, abandoned you. What does that sixteen-year-old say, right now, to his mother?

C: I'm angry, I'm upset. I'm angry with you, mother.

Dr. S.: Yes, again.

C: I'm angry with you. I'm mad that you died and left me. Left me alone. (begins to tear, pause for a minute or two)

Dr. S.: When you look back at that sixteen-year-old, right now, does that boy have any guilt for anything? Were there some things he didn't do or felt he should have done? Does he feel any guilt for having that anger towards his mom, who really loved him and cared for him?

C: Yes, yes. I do have a lot of guilt. I wasn't there for her, when she was sick. I couldn't face it, didn't want to face it.

Dr. S.: How did you feel about that?

C: I'm sad, I'm upset with myself. I should have done more.

Dr. S.: Allow those feelings in.

C: (crying now) I wish I had been there, been there for her.

Dr. S.: Is there sadness? Sadness for the loss, for losing her?

C: Yes, great sadness. (crying more, pause for a minute)

Dr. S.: You miss her. You love her.

C: Yes, very much, very much.

Dr. S.: Can you forgive yourself for not doing as much as you thought you should have? Can you see that this sixteen-year-old boy didn't know what to do, he couldn't deal with the huge loss? He wanted to be there for his mom, but he wasn't able to because he was so young? Can you see that?

C: Yes, that makes sense. I tried, but I was overwhelmed.

Dr. S.: Yes, it was more than you could handle. Can you forgive yourself for that?

C: Yes (crying again), I can.

Dr. S.: Can you say that to yourself?

C: I forgive myself.

Dr. S.: I did the best that I could.

C: I did the best that I could. (sighs, stops crying)

I asked Chris how he felt at this point and he said he was calmer, more relaxed. I explained that by carrying feelings of loss, resentment, guilt and sadness, he was holding onto hurt and pain that continued to affect his mind and body. He felt that a heavy load had been lifted off of his mind by releasing these emotions. After a break, we moved to take on the strong emotions he had towards his father and his father's neglect after the death of his mother.

Dr. S.: After your mom passed away, your father wasn't there for you, was he?

C: No, not at all.

Dr. S.: What did he do?

C: He just buried himself in his work. Never cared about what I was doing, what was going on with me.

Dr. S.: Did he neglect you?

C: Yes, absolutely.

Dr. S.: So, he didn't really care for you then, didn't take care of you, didn't pay attention to you?

C: No, not at all. He just worked and worked.

Dr. S.: What happened to you then?

C: I stopped caring about school, started partying, drinking.

Dr. S.: And then what?

C: I ended up getting kicked out of school. I never recovered that time. I barely graduated from high school, didn't finish college.

Dr. S.: Did you feel that you could have done better?

C: Yes, I was smart, worked hard until…

Dr. S.: When you go back to that time, when you were sixteen, after your mom passed away, when you put yourself in that place, is there any resentment towards your father?

C: Yes, lots.

Dr. S.: Can you express that? What does that sixteen-year-old need to say to his father?

C: I'm angry with you. You weren't there for me.

Dr. S.: You weren't there for me. You didn't care!

C: You didn't care! You just worked and worked.

Dr. S.: I was still your son.

C: I was still your son. What about me?

Dr. S.: You neglected me, never paid attention to me, to my feelings.

C: You neglected me, never paid attention to me!

Dr. S.: I'm furious.

C: I'm furious with you! How could you do that?

Dr. S.: How does your body feel?

C: I want to hurt him.

Dr. S.: Where do you feel this anger, in your body?

C: In my head, my hands.

Dr. S.: If this anger needed to come out, had to come out, right now, what would the anger do? What would the anger do to your father now?

C: It would hit him.

Dr. S.: Where, how?

C: It would punch him in the face.

Dr. S.: Yes, and then what?

C: It would keep punching him, hurting him.

Dr. S.: Would he bleed, get knocked out?

C: Yes, he would be bleeding, fall down.

Dr. S.: Yes, and then what?

C: I would keep hitting him. He would be on the ground.

Dr. S.: Is there still more anger?

C: Yes.

Dr. S.: OK, then what happens?

C: I get on top of him, choke him…he's unconscious. (pause)

Dr. S.: How do you feel now?

C: Still angry.

Dr. S.: So, all the anger's not out yet. What does it do next?

C: It strangles him to death….and then it burns the house down. (takes a deep breath)

Dr. S.: Yes. (pause) How do you feel now?

C: Relaxed, better.

Dr. S.: Do you have any regrets for this treatment of your father?

C: No.

Dr. S.: Do you feel sad for the loss? For losing your father, after you had just lost your mother?

C: Yes, yes, I do. (starts to cry)

Dr. S.: Yes, anyone would. It's very sad, feeling alone, feeling left alone.

C: Yes, it's hurts, it's hard. (crying harder now)

Dr. S.: Let it come, let it all come out.

C: (continues crying, then stops)

Dr. S.: (pauses) Do you notice any sadness for your father? For his loss? He lost his wife, right?

C: Yes, yes. He lost her too. He didn't know what to do. (starts to cry a little)

Dr. S.: You both lost her but couldn't help each other.

C: Yes, we were both hurt. (pause) My dad lost his mother when he was sixteen. (cries harder)

Dr. S.: Yes, lots of hurt, plenty to go around. (pause, crying stops) How do you feel now?

C: Better, calmer.

Dr. S.: Try this. Repeat these wishes out loud: May I be peaceful and contented. (Chris repeats this). May I be free from harm and illness. (Chris repeats). May I be loving and loved. (Chris repeats). May I be forgiving and forgiven. (Chris repeats).

C: I can believe that now.

Dr. S.: How about sending these wishes to your father, right now?

C: Yes, I'd like to do that.

Dr. S.: OK. Repeat these wishes out loud: May he be peaceful and contented. (Chris repeats this). May he be free from harm and illness. (Chris repeats). May he be loving and loved. (Chris repeats). May he be forgiving and forgiven. (Chris repeats).

C: Thank you. I feel much better.

Chris went through a process to open up powerful emotions that had been trapped inside. He was able to access his resentment and anger (towards the loss of his mother and towards the neglect from his father), his guilt (towards how he treated his mother prior to her death), his sadness and grief (for the losses), and his connection and compassion (to his father by recognizing his father's pain and to himself).

Not everyone can access his or her deeper emotions so readily. Not everyone has such powerful feelings for events in their lives. However, everyone has experienced hurtful events and everyone has feelings about those events. The amount of feelings that each person needs to express varies greatly. The feelings of anger or sadness are usually quite uncomfortable and people develop many ways to avoid feeling them. Fear, worry, rationalization, laughter, minimizing or forgetting events, becoming numb, or displacing anger towards others are all ways that the mind avoids strong feelings. These are called defenses and are often helpful at the time when emotional hurts are occurring. They help us cope with stressful events. However, if these defenses become the way we cope with subsequent stressful events and never allow us to recognize and deal with the original emotional hurts, they become part of the problem, rather than part of the solution. Turning anger inward causes guilt, anxiety, depression, and pain. Carrying anger due to an emotional hurt from childhood and expressing it towards people in our current lives doesn't help to resolve the emotional hurt and just perpetuates the problem. EAET allows one to release anger and guilt in order to move towards loving relationships with ourselves and the people in our lives. This model can be used with emotional issues that are current as well as those from the past. The burdens that we carry are the cause of MBS and relieving these burdens allow us to live without anger or guilt and to engage in loving relationships with ourselves and the people in our lives. It also helps teach us to deal with future emotional issues in a way that does not cause MBS symptoms to emerge.

This program presents a variety of methods to recognize deep emotional issues and deal with them. There are cognitive methods, which are ways to think about the issues in your life and investigate how they have affected you. Expressive writing methods are another way that is used to uncover, express, and integrate strong emotions. Finally, there is verbal expression, as demonstrated above. This form of expression is usually done in conjunction with a therapist and if you have access to a therapist who has been trained in ISTDP or EAET, it may be helpful to seek their help. In addition, there are many therapists who use similar methods to get at deep emotions. Willing friends can help people work through the stages of the model as well. In this workbook, I have attempted to describe this model in enough detail to allow individuals to approach this deep emotional work on their own or with a trusted partner. As I have mentioned in the disclaimer at the beginning of this book, please be aware that if you begin to feel overwhelmed with emotions that are difficult to handle, please seek the aid of a counselor. Although the descriptions of this work given here occur in a single session, this work often requires several sessions and often needs to be approached gradually. Nevertheless, I have found that individuals who have the courage to face their life events and their emotions see huge changes in their minds and bodies within minutes when they release long-held feelings. Of course, not everyone with MBS has had significant traumatic life events. Therefore, not everyone will need to do this kind of emotional processing work. In addition, many people who have had trauma may not need to delve into their past in order to recover. But these exercises can be freeing, so don't be afraid. You can proceed gradually and do as much as you are able and willing to do over time. And you can get help as needed.

Memory Reconsolidation

These exercises are based upon recent scientific evidence about memory and the role that emotional memories can play in our lives. Scientists who study memory have learned that our memories are not only often inaccurate, but they are constantly changing (Roemer, et. al., 1998; Schafe, et. al., 2001). This is surprising to most people. When I was young, my brother burned his leg badly and tried to hide it from our parents. I vividly recall seeing him in pain, discovering the burn, and running to get help. The problem with this memory is that it didn't happen that way at all. All of our other family members recall that I had nothing to do with discovering the burn or getting help.

How could I have such a vivid memory of an event (my role in getting help) that never happened?

It turns out that this is an extremely common occurrence. This is why eyewitness accounts of crimes or identification of suspects is often inaccurate. Ten months after a catastrophic airplane crash in the Netherlands, a study found that 55 percent of people reported actually seeing the airplane crash, although no video of the crash existed (Crombag, et. al., 1996). Studies have shown that memories of events shift and alter over time in most people. We remember certain aspects of events or forget other aspects of events as we get older.

Conventional wisdom suggests that we learn to accept that the past is behind us and that we can't change it, and therefore we should try to accept it as it is in order to move forward. This appears to make a lot of sense. However, since your past is merely a summation of your memory of it, and your memory is constantly changing, your past is actually also changing all the time.

Some people who have had traumatic events in their life and continue to have reactions to these events are considered to have post-traumatic stress disorder (PTSD). People with PTSD have outpourings of activity from the autonomic nervous system, which leads to fear and anxiety whenever they recall the traumatic events that triggered the disorder. About a fifth of all combat veterans develop some form of PTSD (Beckham, et. al., 1997). As discussed in chapter 3, there is a very large overlap between PTSD and Mind Body Syndrome. This makes sense, because both PTSD and MBS are triggered by the same kinds of stressful or traumatic events. Furthermore, the brain pathways and structures that activate and perpetuate the symptoms of MBS and PTSD are the same. I consider MBS to be a form of PTSD in which the symptoms tend to be manifest in the body (often with pain), rather than with anxiety. See the companion book, *Unlearn Your Anxiety and Depression*, for a more complete description of this process.

People with PTSD who are successfully treated are those who learn to adapt to their prior traumatic events. One way of accomplishing this is by learning to view and experience their memories differently. They develop ways to make these difficult memories less problematic and easier to accept and cope with. Since our memories are constantly changing and since these memories can affect MBS as well as PTSD symptoms, why not actively work to change our past in ways that allow us to heal and let go of stressful memories? This is precisely what these exercises are designed to accomplish.

This process is known as memory reconsolidation. It is a proven method of going back in time in your imagination to "change" the memories that have been so painful. We do not want you to go back to these memories to simply relive them. That is not helpful at all. Memories exist as packets of information stored in the brain and we reconnect these packets of information into a new or changed story when we go back and think about it. Obviously you cannot change what actually happened. That is not possible. However, this process will guide you to alter these memories in ways that will allow you to picture them in different ways.

If you were treated poorly as a child, it was impossible at that time for you to actually stand up for yourself and stop the mistreatment. But from the vantage point of an adult, you can see that it should have been stopped or changed. By going back in time to that situation in your mind, you can use your imagination and picture changing the story. You can express what needed to be said or you can stop the actions from happening to you. This may seem very odd, silly, or impossible, but it works if you try it. You can also imagine that your current adult self is going back to visit yourself when you were younger and have your adult "help" your younger self to change the memories. You will provide a caring person who offers understanding, compassion, and strength to your younger self who may have felt alone, hurt, abandoned or neglected. Some people have found it useful to bring certain people with them in this process of healing, such as a loving grandparent, friend, or someone who they admire, such as a healer or a religious leader.

There are two meditations that are recorded to accompany this section. Both of them can be found at unlearnyourpain.com, click on the meditations tab at the top of the home page, and use the password, meditations. The first is called Time Traveler and it will guide you through an exercise of visiting your younger self at a difficult time and changing the memories to care for and protect your younger self. You will be guided in this process step by step and you can use it for any situations from your past where you had difficult or hurtful situations.

The second meditation is called Revising the Past, which can be used in conjunction with the Time Traveler meditation. It will guide you to reflect on situations that are from your past, current situations that are difficult, and certain personality traits that you may have in order to treat yourself with compassion and be able to express any emotions that you have and move through them towards health and well-being.

The Process of Emotional Awareness and Expression Therapy

Emotional Awareness and Expression therapy provides a powerful method for dealing with emotions that have been held inside or not fully processed. Remember that you don't necessarily need to engage in EAET. Not everyone will, depending on their particular situation. The key aspects of EAET include actually experiencing the emotions of anger, guilt, and grief (typically in that order) and expressing them fully in order to release them. Because deep-seated resentment and anger underlie most of the issues faced by individuals with MBS, it is important to understand anger and how it can be used as a way to heal.

The key to understanding MBS is the "danger signal" in the brain. In people who have been sensitized by life stresses, the brain can overreact to life events that are not actually dangerous. The danger signal activates a complex series of reactions in the brain and body resulting in pain, anxiety, depression, or other MBS symptoms. Taken as a whole, this is commonly known as the "fight or flight" reaction. The fight or flight reaction is often described as a single, uniform reaction, but fight and flight are separate and different reactions. Both reactions are marked by increased blood flow in the muscles, and they share many other features, but the emotional context is quite different. We run when our primary feeling is fear and we stand and fight when it is anger. In many ways, anger serves to counteract fear. Ongoing fear activates the danger/alarm mechanism, which leads to more pain, anxiety, or depression, while anger leads to feeling powerful, which reduces the danger/alarm mechanism and reduces symptoms.

When someone hurts or abuses us (physically, sexually or emotionally) or when we are injured in some other way, we respond with fear of the hurt/abuse/injury. However, underneath that fear is always some degree of resentment and anger. When the injury is powerful, ongoing and/or occurs early in life, there is often rage towards the offender. This program will help you to release this anger in a direct and therapeutic fashion. However, simply releasing anger in general is neither helpful nor sufficient for healing. Many times, the anger held inside is let out towards people or things who are not the offenders responsible for the anger. Hitting walls or punching pillows isn't healing as an isolated act. Yelling and screaming at friends or family members who were not involved in the original hurt doesn't work. Obviously, people who've been abused in childhood and then go on to abuse others are never acting in useful ways. These are forms of displaced anger; anger that is not directed towards the offender. It only serves to create more problems.

Anger that is directed towards the offender is necessary, but it is important to release that anger in a therapeutic way. Releasing that anger by yelling at the offender in public or punishing or taking revenge on the offender in real life is not a wise course of action and often creates many more problems than it solves. People unfamiliar with EAET often fear that this process will lead to actual violent acts, but this is a misconception. The EAET model allows one to release that anger therapeutically in private. Then one can move on to address the other emotions involved and choose how to act publically in regards to the offender in ways that are wise and useful for the situation.

Getting Started

You can do this work alone or with a partner or therapist. The role of the partner/therapist is to help you to experience the emotions by pushing you towards feeling them and by helping you deflect tendencies to avoid feeling or expressing them. These tendencies are called defenses and everyone uses them. For example, if you ask yourself to focus on the anger and resentment you feel towards someone who harmed you or hurt you, what comes to mind? In order to fully use this model, you need to go directly to that anger. However, we often go to the hurt. "It hurts to think of him" or "I'm afraid when I think of being abused." This is a form of a defense and keeps us in the grips of the offender. Thoughts make up another category of defenses. One may say "It wasn't so bad" or "He didn't mean it" or "Things like that happened in those days." These thoughts serve only to help us avoid the necessary emotion of anger. Another ploy the mind uses is to blame ourselves with phrases like "It was partly my fault" or "I deserved it" or "I should have done something to stop it." These thoughts turn anger inward and are destructive rather than healing. Often the offender is someone whom we love or feel we should love, such as a parent, sibling, other relative, or close friend. In these situations, it is common for our minds to come up with new reasons to avoid anger, such as "I don't want to be angry" or "I don't want to hurt them" or "I've already forgiven them." As should be obvious from the subject of this book, another way to avoid the anger is to develop pain, anxiety and other symptoms in our bodies. When we approach anger towards an offender, our bodies may tighten with pain, we may feel anxious and upset, we may get dizzy or weak or tired, or our minds may have trouble focusing and lose our train of thought. If you notice any of these symptoms, recognize that these are also defenses. It is incredible to see these reactions occur in our bodies; it verifies that MBS symptoms are in fact caused by the mind and its reaction to stressful events in our lives. Finally, acting out, threatening actual violence, or acting violently is another form of a defense from actually feeling the anger and is counterproductive. Actions like this can't heal the emotional hurts from years ago; they serve only to escalate violence and create more misery. It is critical to look for these and any other defenses in order to stop using them. If you allow any of these defenses to take your focus away from feeling the anger, you will not be able to express the anger and heal. Defenses almost always arise, so be on guard to spot them and block them. The goal of EAET is to actually experience the emotions as they were felt in the past and then release them in a therapeutic fashion as described below. Once that occurs, we can act in a way that shows love towards ourselves, is assertive in our actions, protective of ourselves, stops the emotional hurts, and reconciles with those of our choosing. Read this whole section before starting this work.

STEP 1: EXPERIENCING EMOTIONS

Take one of the items on your list from pages 116-118, "List of past traumatic or stressful events." Review the sessions described as a demonstration of what you will be doing. Begin to relive the experience in order to fully feel the emotions that were generated. Do not be afraid of doing this. As I have mentioned, you are not going back to this experience to actually relive it. You are going back to this experience to actually change it. Do not be afraid of feeling strong emotions. Emotions are not harmful; they are necessary and helpful to you. Anger will be present as a way of helping to protect you so that you can be assertive and stand up for yourself. Hurt and sadness are necessary to point you to being compassionate to yourself. Guilt is necessary to help you make amends for any mistakes that you made. Of course, guilt is not necessary or helpful if you are feeling guilt when you did nothing wrong, as we will discuss.

See what emotions arise first when you mentally go back to the situation. If there is resentment or anger, you can proceed to the next section on expressing anger. If there is hurt and sadness, allow those feelings to grow. Place your hand over your heart and feel the sadness and grief. Allow any tears to come out. Do not block these feelings. They will not harm you. I often say that sadness is like a thunderstorm, it is powerful and you will get wet. And, it is necessary to water the earth and it will pass. These feelings are expressions of compassion for you. If you are sad for yourself, it is because you care for yourself. Once the sad feelings have subsided a bit, turn these feelings into kind and caring feelings towards yourself. Breathe in caring and compassion to yourself and to your younger self who was in a difficult situation. Allow these feelings of caring and kindness to flow throughout your body.

Once you have done that, reflect on these questions: Did you deserve to be treated that way? Did you really do anything wrong? Did you deserve better? When you ask these questions, you are guiding yourself towards feelings of self-protection and assertiveness. You are allowing yourself to access feelings of resentment or anger towards how you were treated. Allow those feelings to grow. Do not block them or suppress them. They are important for freeing yourself from these hurts. You are now ready to proceed to the next step.

STEP 2: ALLOWING ANGER TO BE EXPRESSED

Once you are able to actually experience the anger, you are ready to express it. Review the demonstrations. If the stressful events occurred early in life or were very powerful experiences (such as abuse, rape, or other threats to life or body), it is often necessary to have the anger come out in a metaphoric way to attack the offender, such as occurs with Michael or Chris. In the case of situations that occurred later in life, such as with Ed, you may not need the anger to come out in that way; verbal expression of the anger may be enough. In any case, you will know what is necessary by how your body feels as you proceed through this process. When the anger is fully released, you will feel relaxed and calm, or even happy. It is quite an amazing process as you will soon see.

Speak the words that you would have said at the time if you were powerful enough to say anything that should have been said. Be powerful and say whatever comes to your mind to express your anger to the offender. Be strong and honest. Speak out loud. Don't hold anything back. You can scream and yell, be forceful, speak honestly, and use swear words freely in order to help you experience the anger. As you engage in this process, monitor how your body feels and how you are reacting to the feelings of anger. Stop whenever a defense emerges (see the previous section for common defenses) and block it by telling yourself that this is something keeping you from experiencing anger and from healing. If you develop stomach pain or headache or fatigue, recognize that your body is simply reacting to the anger and continue to move into feeling and expressing your anger. Remind yourself that you deserve to be angry, that you were hurt, and that you will not tolerate that or "take it" anymore. Monitor your body for its reaction to the anger. Look for signs that you really feel the anger in your body. You will know that is occurring when you experience the anger in your head and your hands, usually as a warm or hot sensation. It may feel that it is rising up within you. It often helps to clench your fists. Continue this process to allow the anger to well up inside of you. If you begin to feel overwhelmed, stop and rest. Remind yourself that this won't hurt you and that it is a part of your healing process. Then go back and begin again, focusing on the anger, deflecting any defenses that arise, and feeling the anger. This may take several minutes or longer. It may take several different sessions. But this process is very effective as long as you stick with it and do it fully and gradually.

You can always stop for a while and compose yourself before going forward. You can always ask for help from a therapist or counselor. If it is too difficult to express anger out loud, you can write your feelings and allow the anger to "speak" in that way.

After you feel the anger rising up within your body to your hands and head, ask yourself what does the anger need to do to stop the offender, to get back at them, to fully release out of you onto them. The anger may need to be released by physically stopping the offender, not by words, but by acts. Remember that you are not actually doing these acts to them, right now. It is the anger that is doing them and it occurs back at the time of the hurts or abuse. It is healing to allow this anger to be released and it must be released fully. So, ask what would the anger do? You can now describe what happens to the person or people who hurt you, see it happen to them, imagine what the anger does to them. Narrate what happens out loud (or you may choose to write it out in detail on paper). Visualize the scene as you go through it and don't hold anything back. You will probably know when to stop. Do not judge yourself to see if you have expressed "enough" anger. There is usually some kind of relief that you will feel when you are done. You can always come back to this situation to express more feelings later if you need to.

At the end of this process, you will feel better. Your body will relax, your pain will often melt away, and you will feel calmer and freer as though a weight has been lifted off your body. Or, as you will soon see, the anger will turn into guilt or grief. If you continue to feel anger, you may have blocked the process by a defense or by fear. In that case, take a rest and start over later in the day or the next day. Once you have completed this process, you will not need to return to the old feelings of anger. You can finally let them go.

After you have expressed your anger (to whatever extent seems appropriate at this time), take a few moments to purposefully release it. Take some deep breaths. With each breath out, choose to release the anger, gradually, bit by bit. Let it go until you feel calmer. See what emotions arise to replace it, such as any guilt, sadness or compassion, as described in the next sections.

The above examples are dramatic. Many people with MBS have suffered significant trauma in their lives and therefore often have powerful emotions to express. However, almost everyone has had situations in their lives that have caused hurt and emotional pain. As we have seen, not recognizing emotions or holding them in is not generally healthy. The private expression of emotions is something that I believe everyone should learn, even in childhood.

Depending on the level of the hurts, there may a large variation in how much emotion is experienced and therefore how much emotion needs to be expressed. In many of my patients, certain current or past events call for milder expressions of feelings, so do not assume that you will need to express the degree of anger described in the above section. I have worked with many people who needed to express only a much milder degree of either verbal or imagined physical anger. For example, one might need only to say "Back Off!" in a firm way or to imagine simply "shaking" someone in anger. Or it could be an imagined slap on the face or "I just won't take this anymore."

How you feel while doing this work is the key to knowing how much anger needs to be expressed. Some people are able only to access and express a small amount of anger initially. However, when they reflect on their experiences and allow themselves to revisit the hurts, they may still feel significant anger. In that case, they likely need to express more anger more fully. On the other hand, if after expressing the anger in a simple way, there is a feeling of release and relaxation, and there is little anger left upon reflection, that's probably sufficient for the moment. If the anger leads to significant guilt and/or sadness, the process of healing is on track and will result in significant relief of emotional burden and mind-body symptoms if you allow compassion (usually in the form of tears and grief) to soothe the guilt. This step is critical to lift the burden. When these emotions are experienced, most patients feel much lighter, and often pain is reduced or even temporarily eliminated.

This book describes the powerful relationship between pain and emotions. This story illustrates one aspect of this relationship. Edie, a fifty-one-year old woman with back pain, told me with tears in her eyes about the frequent beatings her father gave to her with a belt as a child and teenager. She hid the bruises on her legs by wearing tights. As we discussed her emotional reactions to these beatings, she recalled one episode when she got so angry at her father that, as he was whipping her, she began to yell at him daring him to continue despite her wrath. Amazingly, she noted that she had absolutely no pain while being hit. Her brain had switched from fear to anger, and that turned off the pain response.

STEP 3: LOOK FOR GUILT

As mentioned, there are various forms of guilt that may arise while doing this work. Guilt about having that degree of anger towards a loved one or one that you feel you should love is very common. It is a form of a defense that can prevent the experience and expression of anger. You should realize that everyone has some of this kind of guilt given the emotional or physical hurts that were perpetrated.

Another form of guilt that may arise is the belief that you have done something wrong or that you were in some way responsible for the problems, the situation, or the abuse. While these beliefs are common, they are also usually completely incorrect! When they arise, it is important to examine them critically (often with the help of a trusted friend or therapist) to see them for what they are, which is typically a form of a defense to protect the offenders. This guilt only serves to turn anger inwards. It is destructive to you and you must counteract it. Shame is a particular form of guilt that typically results from not feeling loved and honored as a child. People who feel shame believe that they are not a good or worthy person. Even though these feelings are always incorrect and baseless, if you believe them, it will be more difficult to heal. As an antidote for guilt and shame, repeat these phrases to yourself: "My anger is justified," "I did nothing wrong," "I didn't deserve that treatment," "I am a good person," or "It was not my fault." Take some time to experience the feelings associated with these phrases. They also often lead to tears, which is exactly what you need as you feel these feelings. Even if you truly feel that you actually did something wrong or that you were at fault in some way, it is critically important to forgive yourself. We often find some small thing for which to blame ourselves. In these situations, take time to step back and look at the whole picture. Recognize that your role was probably very small in the overall situation and that the vast majority of the blame deserves to be placed with the offenders. Nevertheless, take time to repeat these phrases: "I was only doing the best I could," "I was caught in a difficult situation," "I was just looking for love," and most importantly, "I forgive myself fully and completely."

STEP 4: EXPERIENCING SADNESS AND GRIEF

In order to complete the experience of processing the emotions that have long been held down, it is useful to look for sadness and grief as well. These feelings often arise spontaneously after releasing the anger and individuals will often simply break into anything from soft tears to powerful sobs. This is a healthy response and what anyone would feel given the difficult situations you have lived through. Allow yourself to feel sadness fully, to experience the grief and regret, and to release these feelings. The words commonly associated with these feelings are "I just wanted to be loved," "I just wanted you to love me," "I was lonely, sad, hurt, or ashamed," "I was afraid," or "I wish things could have been different." Repeat any appropriate phrases as necessary. As described earlier in this section, you can turn the feelings of sadness and grief into feelings of caring and compassion for yourself.

STEP 5: LOVE AND/OR LETTING GO

This is the final step in this process. After experiencing the full range of emotions and releasing them, you are ready to move past the difficult situations of your past. You have taken powerful steps to heal the hurts. When you fully release the anger, guilt, and grief, you won't have to live with those emotions held in any longer. You don't want to harbor anger, guilt, and grief for the rest of your life. These emotions are toxic when kept inside over many years and are responsible for untold suffering from pain, anxiety, fatigue, insomnia, depression, and even substance abuse and other forms of addiction.

This step is to consolidate your emotions and decide how to move forward in real life. When you are able to love yourself, forgive those who can be forgiven and protect yourself from those who continue to be hurtful, you can live in peace and health.

Take some time to practice kindness towards yourself. There are several ways to do this. Here are some suggestions for this step.

- Listen to some of the online meditations each day (available at unlearnyourpain.com, password: meditations).

- Place your hand over your heart. Breathe deeply. Feel your breath filling up your whole body. Breathe in kindness to yourself. Allow feelings of kindness to fill your lungs. Visualize that kindness spreading to every cell and fiber of your body.

- Repeat these phrases: "I am a good person," "I have done the best I could," "I love myself," "I choose to take time for myself," "I deserve to be happy" and any others that make sense to you.

- Repeat these wishes for yourself: "May I be peaceful and contented. May I be free from harm and illness. May I be loving and loved. May I be forgiving and forgiven."

Two excellent books on the subject are *The Mindful Path to Self-Compassion* by Dr. Christopher Germer and *Self-Compassion* by Dr. Kristin Neff. These books have several exercises to enhance compassion towards self and others. You can repeat some of these exercises on a regular basis while you are completing the program in this book.

After taking time to experience feelings of kindness and compassion for yourself, you are ready to decide how to act towards others in real life. There are two main categories of people in your life: those whom you choose to forgive and love and those whom you need to avoid, set boundaries with, and protect yourself from. And there are those who fall in the middle between these extremes.

There may be people who have hurt you, yet you can forgive them and continue to have a relationship with them. Often these are parents or siblings who have changed or mellowed over the years. If they are not hurting you now, you may be able to have a loving relationship with them going forward. If you have let go of the old hurts and the anger, you may be able to forgive them or at least let go of the past. For these people, it is often helpful to take time to send them wishes of kindness and choose to develop a new way of being with them.

Repeat these wishes for them: "May they be peaceful and contented. May they be free from harm and illness. May they be loving and loved. May they be forgiving and forgiven."

On the other hand, there are people who were offenders and are not part of your life, or you do not want them to be in your life. For these people, you need to "let go" of them. You cannot allow them to hurt you anymore. You need to avoid them or set boundaries on how you choose to relate to them. Common examples would be a rapist or another offender who chooses to continue to be hurtful in words or deeds. For these people, you will need to act assertively and forcefully to protect yourself. However, you do not want to act violently or aggressively. Hopefully, you have released your anger towards them in the process described above. If you continue to feel anger towards them, you may need to repeat the process above to more fully rid yourself of the anger.

You can repeat phrases such as these: "You can't hurt me anymore," "I'm through with you," "I won't allow you to hurt me anymore," "I will protect myself from you," "I will set boundaries and not allow you to cross them," or "I love myself enough to not be hurt by you again." You can say these forcefully and with assertiveness.

It can be helpful to reflect on some of these people. Often, they are very flawed individuals and they may also be suffering from hurts of their own. Most people don't act to hurt others unless they are also hurting. This doesn't forgive what they did or excuse it. However, some people have been able to find some degree of caring or even pity for those who hurt them. They may not have acted appropriately or civilly, but it may have been the best that they were able to do under the circumstances. Being able to express some degree of kindness to these people can be a part of your healing journey to move forward with your life and let go of the past.

If these people are not part of your life, you can fully let go of their hurts and their influence over you. You are definitely through with them and they cannot hurt you anymore. For those who continue to be part of your life, such as an ex-spouse, decide how you will act when you encounter them. You can choose to leave your anger behind, yet be strong enough to create terms of a relationship that suit you and allow your needs to be met as much as possible. You will often need to set boundaries in order to protect yourself. You may need to discuss these issues with a trusted friend or therapist to choose the best possible options.

I have outlined a step-by-step EAET process, but be flexible in how you approach and complete this work. For example, the first emotions that arise when examining a traumatic issue are often grief and sadness, not resentment and anger. Allow those feelings to come up, and feel them fully. Letting the physical sensations of grief well up in your heart and letting tears of sadness flow are important parts of the healing process. You may then be able to open yourself up to other feelings, such as resentment. As mentioned, there is almost always some degree of resentment—which can range up to anger or rage—for situations in which we were hurt. It's important to feel and express that. And there is often guilt, either for the anger one feels or as part of shame and self-blaming. Expressing that guilt and remorse is also important for healing. No matter what order the emotions are accessed and experienced, the important work is to feel them, accept them as being normal and healthy, express them, and release them.

I have found the following exercise to be of great benefit. It can begin the EAET process or complete it. It helps to access compassion for self, which is a critical aspect of recovery from MBS. This process is fully described in the Time Traveler meditation at unlearnyourpain.com, password: meditations. Begin by going back in time to review moments when you felt hurt, abused, neglected, or abandoned in some way, or simply in need of love and caring. Take a few deep breaths and close our eyes to allow you to look back to your younger self. Allow yourself to feel for your younger self; allow feelings of kindness, compassion, and caring for your younger self to arise. Picture yourself putting your arm around the shoulder of your younger self or holding her or him. Picture your younger self feeling the caring and compassion you are giving. Speak to your younger self out loud or silently with kindness and caring. You may say things such as, "You are a good person. You didn't do anything wrong. You didn't deserve to be treated that way. You will be OK. You will get through this, and you will come out OK. I will love you. You are now safe, and I will protect you. I will care for you, and you are not alone." See if your younger self can hear those words and feel your touch. See if your younger self can begin to relax in that time and place. You may feel a relaxation in your body as tension reduces. Allow yourself a few moments to feel the compassion and sense of safety that arises. These feelings help to reset your brain from the "fight or flight" reaction to one of security and peacefulness, which reverses neural pathways of pain, anxiety, and depression. Since you carry that younger self with you, healing that self's hurts also heals yours.

You can repeat this exercise several times in order to develop new neural circuits of safety and compassion. You can do this for any situation of past hurt. Doing so reinforces neural pathways that will be more likely to be accessed automatically in the future.

You can increase the healing benefit of this exercise by going a step farther with this visualization.

Once the younger self begins to feel better, she or he can then return the favor by giving caring messages to your current self. See if you can imagine a stronger, more secure version of your younger self speaking to your current self, saying something like: "You are a great person. I am feeling better now, and you can too. You don't need to worry about me. I'll be OK. And now you can be OK too. Love yourself and take care of yourself. You will be fine."

Finally, you can do another exercise to increase self-compassion, which is commonly in short supply for many people. Picture someone who you love unconditionally, such as a spouse, parent, sibling, or child. Imagine offering love and caring for that person. Allow yourself to feel those feelings completely. Now imagine that person giving you similar offerings of kindness, caring, and love. Allow yourself to feel those feelings coming back to you. Take some deep breaths and experience those caring feelings going back and forth between you and your loved one. Realize that as someone who can love, you are also deserving of receiving those feelings in return. Thank yourself for being kind and caring. Allow yourself to accept the fact that you are a good person, someone who tries to do the right thing, and someone who deserves to be happy. Take some more deep breaths and allow yourself to stay in this moment as you accept yourself and practice being kind to yourself.

If you are unsure of how to proceed in your life, especially in relation to certain relationships, you might try this exercise. Sit in a comfortable spot and close your eyes. Think of someone whom you hold in great esteem. It could be someone who have known in your life, such as a parent, grandparent or teacher or someone who is a great leader or wise person, such as a religious leader, political leader, educator or healer. Imagine that person or entity is paying you a visit, taking time to sit with you and listen to your situation. Tell them what they need to know and ask for their advice on how to handle it and how to proceed. Imagine what they would tell you, what advice they would give and what words they would use. Listen carefully and see how you might apply this wisdom in your life. Thank them for the visit and suggest that you may call on them again in the future as necessary. Take some deep breaths and allow your eyes to open.

Using the Emotional Worksheets As You Complete this Program

The lists you have completed on pages 116-118 will serve as a guide. I suggest that you use the EAET framework as described above with several of the items on those lists. You can decide which ones need to be done. As you go through them, you may find that some of them do not need to be addressed in this way. After doing this emotional work, you can complete the emotional worksheets as described below as a way of reflecting on the work you have done and moving past these emotional issues by letting them go and deciding what actions you may need to take in your life (if any) to move forward.

Here are some examples of ways to complete the worksheets.

Issue: Physical and emotional abuse by my ex-husband _____

Anger/Resentment: I've expressed my anger towards him and "killed" him in my mind

_____

Guilt/Shame: It was not my fault, but I feel I could have left him earlier; I forgive myself for this as I wanted to try to keep the family together as long as I could _____

_____

Sadness/Grief: I've expressed my sadness in tears _____

Love/Letting go: I love myself, I forgive him, but I will protect myself from him so he can't hurt me anymore _____

Lessons learned: I will only enter into new relationships that are not abusive_____

Actions: I will act with civility towards him, but set boundaries on how often I see him and speak to him; If he acts aggressively, I will immediately stop the conversation and leave

_____

Issue: My boss is controlling and micromanaging _____

Anger/Resentment: I have expressed my anger towards him (privately) and have released it; I know I will not change him _____

Guilt/Shame: I feel no guilt about my anger towards him; I have done nothing wrong and have no shame _____

Sadness/Grief: It is sad that I do not enjoy my work as much as I could _____

Love/Letting go: I love myself, I let go of my dependence on his approval, and I will protect myself from his controlling ways _____

Lessons learned: There are many bosses like him and I hope to get a different one soon
_____

Actions: I will go to work each day with a positive attitude, and apply for different jobs this year _____

1. Issue: _____
    Anger/Resentment: _____
    Guilt/Shame: _____
    Sadness/Grief: _____
    Love/Letting go: _____
    Lessons learned: _____
    Actions: _____

2. Issue : _____

     Anger/Resentment:_____

     Guilt/Shame :_____

     Sadness/Grief: _____

     Love/Letting go: _____

     Lessons learned: _____

     Actions: _____

3. Issue: _____

     Anger/Resentment:_____

     Guilt/Shame: _____

     Sadness/Grief: _____

     Love/Letting go: _____

     Lessons learned: _____

     Actions: _____

4. Issue: _____

     Anger/Resentment:_____

     Guilt/Shame:_____

     Sadness/Grief: _____

     Love/Letting go: _____

     Lessons learned: _____

     Actions:_____

5. Issue: _____

     Anger/Resentment:_____

     Guilt/Shame: _____

     Sadness/Grief: _____

     Love/Letting go: _____

     Lessons learned: _____

     Actions:_____

6. Issue: _____

      Anger/Resentment:_____

      Guilt/Shame: _____

      Sadness/Grief: _____

      Love/Letting go: _____

      Lessons learned: _____

      Actions:_____

Writing Exercise for Week Three: Dialogues

A dialogue is basically a conversation that you create in a written form. The writing exercise for this week is in the form of a dialogue. In a dialogue, you have the opportunity to express yourself to someone (or some entity), and to hear some things that you may need to hear from the other person or entity. One reason for writing these dialogues is to gain insight and learn more about important issues in your life. Dialogues may help you better understand situations that are confusing to you or those about which you need to make important decisions. Some of the dialogues may be short, ten-minute jottings, while others may be longer pieces that you return to again and again to explore whatever you need to explore regarding a relationship you have with a part of yourself or another. Dialogues offer insights into important issues in our lives when they tap into wisdom that comes from our inner knowing. When we engage in a dialogue from our heart, we can say what needs to be said and hear what we need to hear.

The first step is to make a list of possible dialogues you might create. You may need to dialogue with a parent, another relative, a current or former spouse, significant other, friend, neighbor, colleague, boss, or coworker. You may choose to dialogue with someone who has died or a person from whom you are estranged, as well as with people who are present in your life today. You can dialogue with people whom you've never met, with religious leaders, political figures, or even God. Some of these may be recipients of unsent letters, but there are other entities that you might want to consider dialoguing with. For example, you may want to "converse" with one or more body parts that are causing you discomfort. You could dialogue with parts of your subconscious mind, such as the internal parent (who may push you to do all the things you "should" do) or the internal child (who may become angry or afraid). Another group of dialogues can be written with personality traits that you've learned, such as the worrying self, the self-critical self, or the overly conscientious or perfectionist self. It is often very helpful to write a dialogue with yourself at an earlier age, such as at a time in your life that was particularly difficult or stressful. Or you may choose to write a dialogue between yourself now and yourself at some point in the future, when you have recovered from MBS. You may choose to dialogue with an event or situation in its entirety, not just a person involved in it. You can even dialogue with a business or an institution. Use your imagination, and be creative. If there is someone or something that is causing you stress in your life, you can write an imaginary dialogue and see what you can learn in order to help ease your mind or figure out how to better deal with it.

Many people have found that it's useful to create a dialogue between yourself and your symptom, whether it's pain, anxiety, depression, insomnia, or fatigue. You can learn a lot by having such a conversation. If you start the dialogue with an open mind, ask simple questions and listen to the answers, you often learn some important things. Sometimes the symptom tells you to let go of some issue or to stop blaming yourself, or to make some change in your life. You can ask what the symptom needs to stop bothering you. This dialogue may not work every time, but it's worth trying; it may lead to a significant boost in your recovery.

Consider all of these factors and any of the exercises you've done so far in this program and create a list of possible people or entities that you would like to engage in dialogue. Use the space provided to compile a list.

My list of possible dialogues includes:

_____

_____

_____

_____

_____

_____

_____

_____

_____

_____

_____

_____

_____

_____

_____

_____

Select Those Dialogues You Think Might Prove Most Beneficial

During this week, you will be choosing a person or entity each day for a dialogue. Take a look at your list now, and circle the ones that you think might be most helpful for you to write first. Once you begin writing, you may discover you need to continue a dialogue for more than one day with the same person or thing. Feel free to do this as necessary. Once you see what you need to learn or express, you can move on to dialogue with other people or entities.

Some people have found it helpful to dialogue with a group (as if creating a meeting or conference call). For example, you could dialogue with yourself, your pain, and your subconscious mind.

Getting a Dialogue Started

When you write, feel free to allow your mind and hand to write whatever needs to be said to the person, situation, or entity you've chosen to address. Since the dialogue will remain on paper, you can say anything that comes to your mind without censoring what you write.

A good way to begin a dialogue is by writing a simple statement or a question. See what response might arise. Let your mind, your heart, and your hand go in whatever direction they will. Allow the person, situation, or entity to respond with whatever comes into your mind about how they might respond. It is important to be able to listen to what arises. Many people have found that they need to learn something from others in their life or from their pain or symptoms.

These are obviously imaginary dialogues, and you won't know exactly what responses might occur in real life. Don't script these dialogues ahead of time, but rather allow them to unfold as they occur. If you allow yourself to fully engage in the imaginary dialogues, you will often uncover hidden truths and learn something about yourself and your life circumstances. You will be better able to move past MBS.

Most dialogues take about ten to fifteen minutes, but you can write as long as you need to. After each dialogue, write your affirmations in the space provided.

Letters to Yourself

After writing your dialogues this week, reflect on and write a description of what you have learned. This may include what you have learned from this person, event, or entity and in what ways you can see that you may have grown as a result of your relationship with him, her, or it. State how you've been able to deal with any issues related to the subject of your dialogue and how you plan on dealing in the future with any issues that have come to your attention or have been left behind from the past. See Progoff for more on dialogues (1975).

Week Three, Day One:

Identify who the speakers will be below and then write a dialogue chosen from the list. It is helpful to continue to write the name of each speaker preceding what he, she, or it says. Express your thoughts and feelings fully. Use as much paper as needed. Remember to allow the other person, event, or entity to respond to you fully as well.

Speaker 1 = _____

Speaker 2 = _____

The Dialogue

Reflect on the dialogue you wrote in a letter to yourself or to someone else. What have you learned from this dialogue? In what ways have you gained from this interaction (even if there were very negative aspects of the relationship)? How have you been able to deal with any issues related to this relationship, and how do you plan on dealing with these issues in the future?

Dear _____,

Week Three, Day Two:

Create a dialogue in the space below.

Speaker 1 = _____

Speaker 2 = _____

The Dialogue

Reflect on the dialogue you wrote in a letter to yourself or to someone else.

Dear _____,

Week Three, Day Three:

Create a dialogue in the space below.

Speaker 1 = _____

Speaker 2 = _____

The Dialogue

Reflect on the dialogue you wrote in a letter to yourself or to someone else.

Dear _____,

Week Three, Day Four:

Create a dialogue in the space below.

Speaker 1 = _____

Speaker 2 = _____

The Dialogue

Reflect on the dialogue you wrote in a letter to yourself or to someone else.

Dear _____,

Week Three, Day Five:

Create a dialogue in the space below.

Speaker 1 = _____

Speaker 2 = _____

The Dialogue

Reflect on the dialogue you wrote in a letter to yourself or to someone else.

Dear _____,

Week Three, Day Six:

Create a dialogue in the space below.

Speaker 1 = _____

Speaker 2 = _____

The Dialogue

Reflect on the dialogue you wrote in a letter to yourself or to someone else.

Dear _____,

Week Three, Day Seven:

Create a dialogue in the space below.

Speaker 1 = _____

Speaker 2 = _____

The Dialogue

Reflect on the dialogue you wrote in a letter to yourself or to someone else.

Dear _____,

An Internal Family Systems Approach: A Special Type of Dialogue Writing

Internal family systems (IFS) is a therapeutic approach that was developed by Richard Schwartz (Schwartz, 2020). It recognizes what most people intuitively understand, that we are made up of different parts. For example, one part of us is excited about new opportunities, while the other part is fearful of change. One part of us works hard to achieve, while another part criticizes us as being a loser. One part of us feels obligated to care for an aging parent, while the other part resents doing it since that parent may not have been supportive when we were younger. These parts represent normal divisions that arise over the course of a lifetime, but are particularly important to understand in those who are dealing with chronic pain, anxiety and depression.

Many of these parts develop or become stronger in response to stressful life events that cause our brain to feel endangered. They are often a coping mechanism or a way for our brain to protect us from the effects of those events. For example, if you were criticized by a parent, you may develop a strong internal critic that protects you from being anything less than perfect to avoid more criticism. A whole category of these protectors can serve to manage your life by keeping you as safe as possible. These so-called "managers" are traits like perfectionism, internal criticism, putting others first, never standing out, overworking, not letting others get close to us, and feeling insecure and needy. Many people live their lives this way, which sets them up for MBS when new significant stressors occur. At these times, if we feel particularly threatened and our brains really feel endangered, other protectors, known as "firefighters" may take over. These are protectors that are so powerful that they literally take over our lives for some amount of time. They can cause us to be incapable of normal functioning. These may include binge drinking or drug use, sexual promiscuity, self-harm and thoughts of suicide, or severe pain, anxiety or depression. You can see that from an IFS perspective, MBS symptoms are simply different manifestations of protectors. When you get bouts of headaches, abdominal or pelvic discomfort, dizziness, tinnitus, back pain or other symptoms, your brain is sending a message that there is some danger. Your brain is not betraying you, it is trying to protect you.

It is tempting to view these firefighters as the problem we need to fix. We desperately want to stop drinking, self-harm, anxiety, depression and pain; we want to see these conditions as the problem. The symptoms are usually so bothersome and worrisome that we tend to react to them with what I call the six Fs: fear of them, focus on them, fighting with them, frustration with them, trying to figure them out, and trying to fix them. Unfortunately, all of these reactions tend to create increased pressure on ourselves, which leads to an increase in the danger/alarm mechanism thus creating even more pain and other symptoms.

However, when we recognize that these protectors are simply different parts of us, we can examine them, understand them, and learn from them. We can see that these conditions are actually the solution that your brain has devised. Therefore, what we really need to do is to see these as neural circuits in the brain and realize that the best way to recover is to get to the underlying causes. In other words, to view the symptoms of chronic pain, anxiety and depression as protectors, as messengers of sorts, as a barometer of an underlying situation.

The IFS model leads to particularly effective treatments as it recognizes and deals with the internal conflicts that are present. It points out that the protectors are covering up some kind of internal hurt or insecurity or emotional reaction that needs to be identified, explored and processed. The process of IFS involves getting to know the protectors and viewing them as helpful parts, rather than problems to get rid of. You can create a dialogue with a protector, such as the internal critic or the pain itself, in order to have it identify the underlying issues and process them. You can use the dialogue writing model described below to accomplish this.

Pick a protector, such as your pain or other MBS symptom. Start with a question that you ask yourself. How do you feel towards this protector? Make a short list of your feelings towards this protector. Often your reactions towards this protector are feelings such as the 6 Fs listed above.

Since the goal of this exercise is to get to learn from the protector and let it help you, each of these negative reactions towards the protector will get in the way of further understanding. Therefore for each of these reactions, you can ask the reaction to kindly step aside for a few minutes in order to allow you to interact directly with the protector in a more understanding and helpful way. Let these protectors know that you honor them and appreciate how they are trying to protect you.

Now that you are able to set aside the negative reactions to MBS symptoms, please write another short list of positive ways that you feel towards MBS. Hopefully, you will get to a place where you can view the protector with curiosity, calmness, and even compassion. When this occurs, you are ready to learn from the pain, anxiety or depression and to ask it to help you.

Now start a written dialogue with the symptom. Ask it these questions: What message do you have for me? What specifically are you protecting me from? What are you afraid would happen to me if you didn't take over my life? At what point in my life did you begin? How old was I? What was happening at that time?

The answers to these crucial questions will help you understand why you have these symptoms. They will likely lead you to some underlying hurts and emotions that are at the core of the pain. For example, the pain may be protecting you from hurts that are occurring currently in your life at work or in your family. You might find that a certain situation threatens to make you feel very small or invisible, or to feel great guilt or shame.

If your symptom points towards a current life situation, begin a dialogue in writing between that part of you that feels upset or threatened or shamed. Ask it what you need to know and see about the situation. Tell that part of you that you see it, hear it and understand it. Tell it that you care for it and that you will act to help it not feel so bad. Tell it that you will promise to try to not put yourself in situations that cause this part to feel this way. Ask this part if it hears you and can begin to trust you. See how you feel after doing this dialogue.

If the situation that you become aware of happened some time ago, create a written dialogue with that younger version of yourself, using these questions: What does this younger version of yourself need to tell you about this situation? What do you need to see that happened so you can witness the event with your caring and compassionate adult eyes? What does your adult caring self need to do to help the younger version of yourself? That younger version may need you to go to them, soothe them, or care for them. He/she may need you to rescue them, protect them from a dangerous person, fight back for them, or speak out for them. He/she may need you to take them away, get them to a safe place, or to a happier place, where they can enjoy themselves. Write out in vivid detail how these events can now occur in your mind's eye. Write out how you witness and care for your younger self, how you protect your younger self, how you stand up for them, and how you take them away to a safe and even an enjoyable place.

In this way, you can heal some of the hurts that lead to MBS. After doing this, you can continue the dialogue with your younger self to see how the younger version of yourself feels now. You can ask if your younger self is ready to let go of the hurts and emotions that have persisted for so long. For example, you can ask your younger self if they want to put those feelings and those experiences in a box, or burn them in a fire or release them into the air. If you do that, see how you feel at this point. You may feel lighter as you let go of troublesome events from the past.

You can repeat this exercise with any issues that have been causing emotional pain. It is a powerful model for relieving held hurts, even if they have been there for a long time. You can learn more about IFS or find therapists who are trained in IFS at selfleadership.com.

Meditation for Week Three: Dialogue with the Subconscious Mind

You will find another meditation for this week at unlearnyourpain.com, click on the meditations tab at the top, and use the password, meditations. The theme concerns a dialogue and fits in with the change in tone for this week's exercises. You will be moving towards an integration of your mind and body, having them work together for health and happiness. Begin this dialogue with your mind in the spirit of cooperation and harmony.

Meditation Synopsis

Find a spot where you will not be disturbed for several minutes. Start with the basic breathing techniques of noticing each breath, accepting it as it is, and letting each breath go. Notice that the subconscious mind is made up of everything that has occurred in the past, everything that is currently happening, and how it has reacted to these events. Recognize that the subconscious has a child-mind component and a parent-mind component. Recognize that the subconscious is not always rational, yet we are able to communicate with it. Gently ask the subconscious mind to stop causing the physical symptoms and emotional reactions that have occurred in the past. Tell the subconscious mind that you understand that it has been upset or hurt, but that you do not want to be in pain. Tell the subconscious child-mind that you will pay attention to it, but that you will not tolerate the development of any physical symptoms. Tell the subconscious parent-mind that you will pay attention to it, but that you will not tolerate the production of any physical symptoms. Picture the subconscious mind as a sea with rippling currents and small waves. When you instruct the subconscious to stop causing symptoms, picture the sea turning calm and quiet.

Picture your body as healthy. Picture every body part as functioning normally, able to participate in daily life without any significant pain or discomfort. Thank the subconscious mind for allowing the symptoms to diminish and disappear. Tell the subconscious that you will pay attention to it in the future so there is no real need for it to cause these symptoms to occur. Repeat to yourself three times, "I fully and completely accept myself. I let go of issues that have bothered me in the past. I choose to respond to my current stressors so they don't affect my health. I realize that I am not perfect, but I choose to accept my personality as it is, and I will not let any of these issues affect my health. I take pride in doing this work, which helps me to be in control and to be more healthy in mind and body."

Reprogramming the Brain: Pain Reprocessing continued

The pain reprocessing techniques for this week focus on becoming more accepting of yourself. Now, you can gently remind your brain that these symptoms are no longer necessary. You can gently laugh at yourself and at how the mind creates some of the symptoms. You can make friends with yourself and your subconscious mind. The goal is to be whole and at peace with yourself. Work at being loving and accepting of yourself, and that includes accepting your internal child, your internal parent, your conscious mind, and your subconscious mind. Recognize that you're not perfect and that you may still continue to have MBS symptoms at times (I certainly do), but the more you can be kind to yourself and the more you can love and accept your whole self, the better you'll be able to fend off physical and psychological symptoms and become healthier and happier.

Another thing you can do is to reward your subconscious mind for "good" behavior. This, of course, is a classic way to retrain or reprogram. We are going to start using the "carrot" with the subconscious mind. Think of ways you can reward yourself and your subconscious mind. Make sure to thank the subconscious mind for getting better. Praise it, and tell it that it's doing a great job by letting go of old patterns and by learning new ones. Do more things that you enjoy. You will be rewarding yourself and your mind, and you will feel more whole as you make peace within yourself.

So, this week, work at being kind to yourself. When you talk to your mind and your body, speak more gently and laugh if you can at certain situations and triggers that produce symptoms. When you catch yourself having MBS symptoms, it can be similar to catching a beloved child with his hand in the cookie jar. You can chuckle at the child because he doesn't mean to be naughty; he was just trying to get away with something. You can correct it in a loving, positive way, as you would a child, knowing that you accept the subconscious as part of you and that it will learn.

One man who went through this program had these words of wisdom.

"The acceptance tip is as follows; when you feel the pain, simply and gently say "thinking" to yourself. All pain exists in the brain. Condition your brain, that the pain is only that, a thought. Then return to what you were doing.

You may have to do this 100s or even 1000s of times, but eventually your brain will become bored of this game. You really don't care how many times you have to do this, because you don't put a healing timetable on your pain. Why would you? You have already completely accepted it as a thought that can't hurt you."

I had a patient who had a history of neck and shoulder pain for several years. After seeing me, he made a realization: that he wasn't actually damaged or injured physically and that basically, he was OK and that he was going to be OK. Over the next several weeks, he used one simple intervention: he told himself that he was OK. During each day, he found time to say: "Robbie, you're OK," over and over. Gradually, over time, he felt better and better. After a couple of months, his pain was gone.

Finally, you must realize that MBS symptoms are fueled by the attention that we give them. The more we are preoccupied with the symptom, the more it has our attention and the more it thrives. When we continuously think about the pain, worry about it, and fear it, the more it is reinforced and engrained in our brain and body. It is often extremely difficult to stop thinking about pain or other symptoms. However, it is necessary to cut off the fuel to the pain. So, you must retrain yourself to be less worried, less afraid of, and less preoccupied with the pain. When you find yourself doing any of those things, you have to stop it, let go of those thoughts and relax. Turn your mind to something else. One way to accomplish this is to "change the channel" in the brain. Many people have found it helpful to simply start doing something else. One patient found that turning on music and dancing vigorously was very effective. Singing or reciting something out loud can be useful. Participating in a physical activity, such as swinging a golf club, kicking a soccer ball, or knitting can literally change the focus of your mind off the pain. Engage fully in the new activity and allow your mind to focus on that instead of the pain. Of course, you want to do this activity knowing full well that there is nothing wrong with you, that you are healthy and strong, and that you can learn to stop your pain and other MBS symptoms.

A useful way to think about retraining your brain is to think of yourself as your own coach.

A good coach knows players or students need both praise and gentle pushing to do more and do better. Sometimes they need a firm reminder to work harder, and sometimes they need a supportive presence to calm them and help them see how far they've come and what their potential is. While working on ridding yourself of chronic pain, anxiety, depression, or other symptoms, you are like an athlete learning a sport. You must believe in yourself and be optimistic you can improve. It helps to have a coach who believes in you. Be your own coach. Athletes also need someone to push them to do more and take risks, and your own inner coach can give you the courage to take on your symptoms and push yourself to be more active, even if you have pain or other symptoms. Challenge yourself as a good coach would do to try new activities and move forward. Take time to praise yourself. A helpful motto is "Great job, now try this."

I also want to warn you about a common problem that may arise while working on this program. As I have pointed out earlier, many people with MBS are exceptionally hardworking and perfectionistic. They often put a lot of pressure on themselves and have high expectations for themselves. They may tend to criticize themselves. If they are unable to do every bit of homework in this program, they often begin to get down on themselves, which only makes matters worse. They may believe that they won't get better unless they complete every assignment. Do not fall into this trap. Few people complete each and every assignment, yet most people get better. Do as much as you feel you need to do or can do within the constraints of your daily life.

As a gentle reminder, we want to treat our brain as if we were training a puppy. You may have developed MBS over many months or years and you may have had these symptoms for a long time. It may take some time to reprogram your brain so that your brain feels safe and turns off the MBS symptoms. I want to remind you that if you are putting pressure on yourself to recover quickly, if you are putting a timetable on your recovery, if you are desperately hoping that your symptoms will just magically disappear, then you are actually making it harder to recover. It is important to keep doing the work contained in this book and trust that you will get better. If you can focus on living your best life, instead of focusing on your symptoms, you will get better; and you may even find that your recovery occurs without you being aware of it. When you practice patience, trust, and compassion for yourself, you are altering the neural circuits of MBS.

Rebuilding Your Life: Make Commitments to Yourself

This week I invite you to engage in some specific activities that will help you in your recovery from MBS. You probably need to break some habits that have held you back. Many people are limited in what physical activities they do because of pain or fear of pain. In order to cure yourself, you will need to face these issues head-on and start to overcome them. Choose some activities to free yourself and move your recovery forward.

Choose to do some things that will make you happy. If you rarely do anything for yourself, it may be somewhat difficult to find things to do, but it is important that you act. Also, find some things to do for others, not out of obligation, but things that will also give you pleasure.

Finally, choose only those activities that you believe are most important to you and those that you believe you can actually carry out. Make a list of those activities on the next page. List those things you are willing to make a commitment to doing.

Exercise: Things I Make a Commitment to Doing

Activities:

This week:

In the next month:

In the next six months to one year:

Things for myself:

This week:

In the next month:

In the next six months to one year:

Things for others:

This week:

In the next month:

In the next six months to one year:

Act on Your Commitments:

Now take the items in the above lists **that pertain to this week** and begin to plan for completing them. Take the ones that might be more difficult to accomplish, and use the following worksheets to help you figure out how to do them.

Worksheet for planning and carrying out commitments:

List the action _____

When do you plan on starting it? When do you plan on achieving it? _____
_____
_____

How will you accomplish it? What steps do you need to take? Which ones will you do first?
_____
_____
_____
_____
_____
_____

What kind of help or aid will you need? Who can help you? What strategies will you need to use to achieve your goals? _____
_____
_____
_____
_____

What barriers might you encounter? How will you overcome them? _____
_____
_____
_____

I make a commitment to this activity by _____ (date).

Signed _____

Worksheet for planning and carrying out commitments:

List the action _____

When do you plan on starting it? When do you plan on achieving it? _____

_____

_____

How will you accomplish it? What steps do you need to take? Which ones will you do first?

_____

_____

_____

_____

_____

What kind of help or aid will you need? Who can help you? What strategies will you need to use to achieve your goals? _____

_____

_____

_____

_____

What barriers might you encounter? How will you overcome them? _____

_____

_____

_____

_____

I make a commitment to this activity by _____ (date).

Signed _____

Worksheet for planning and carrying out commitments:

List the action _____

When do you plan on starting it? When do you plan on achieving it? _____

_____

_____

How will you accomplish it? What steps do you need to take? Which ones will you do first?

_____

_____

_____

_____

_____

What kind of help or aid will you need? Who can help you? What strategies will you need to use to

achieve your goals? _____

_____

_____

_____

_____

What barriers might you encounter? How will you overcome them? _____

_____

_____

_____

_____

I make a commitment to this activity by _____ (date).

Signed _____

chapter 10

Week Four:
Creating the New You

Seize the very first possible opportunity to act on every resolution you make, and on every emotional prompting you may experience in the direction of habits you aspire to gain. — William James

Even though you may want to move forward in your life, you may have one foot on the brakes. In order to be free, we must learn how to let go. Release the hurt. Release the fear. Refuse to entertain your old pain. The energy it takes to hang onto the past is holding you back from a new life. What is it you would let go of today? — Mary Manin Morrissey

How do you feel about yourself? If you're like most people, you have a variety of positive and negative thoughts about yourself, ranging from kind to disparaging. The way you talk to yourself can have great effects on how you are and what you do. You can choose how you see yourself and which aspects you emphasize in yourself. And once you begin to act in ways that emphasize the qualities you admire in yourself, those actions become habits that are easier to perform regularly. The more you act in ways that are consistent with how you'd like to be, your self-image changes.

If you want to be kinder to yourself or to your family, you can practice being kinder in small ways on a regular basis. If you want to be more assertive, practice saying "no" when asked to do something that you really don't want to do. If you want to be more generous or more outgoing, you can practice acting in those ways. If you want to be healthier, more active, or more fit, you can begin to do things that make you this way, and you will come to see yourself as a healthier, more active, and more fit person.

A good first step is to look inward to discover some positive qualities that you often ignore. There is an old story about a Native American elder who is telling his grandson about two creatures who are at war inside him: one a wild dog that is mean, vicious, and tells lies; the other an eagle that is kind, just, and honest. The small boy's eyes widen, and he asks his grandfather who will win this war. The elder statesman answers: "Whichever one I feed."

It is up to you to notice this "war" that occurs in you. You can choose to "feed"—to pay attention to and nourish—those qualities that move you in the direction you would like to travel. You can choose to live in anger, fear, guilt, and sadness, or you can live in love, hope, and joy. You make these choices daily. The more often you choose to live in love, hope, and joy, the more that will be who you are.

Writing Exercises for Week Four

Gratitude List

When you are in pain for any significant length of time, the pain or anxiety or depression or other symptoms can often become all that you think about. These symptoms, thoughts about them, and feelings about them, can easily take over your life to the point where there is nothing left. In order to rid yourself from these symptoms, you need to be able to pay attention to the things in your life that are working and that are good. One step in this direction is to give thanks for the positives in your life.

Make a list of things for which you are grateful. Include anything you can think of—such as having a roof over your head, food to eat, the sun rising each day, a color, friends, family, etc. Consider including things for which you may be only partly grateful, for example, difficult people or things that may have taught you important lessons.

Gratitude List:

a. _____

b. _____

c. _____

d. _____

e. _____

f. _____

g. _____

h. _____

i. _____

j. _____

k. _____

l. _____

m._____

n. _____

o. _____

p. _____

q. _____

r. _____

s. _____

t. _____

u. _____

v. _____

w._____

x. _____

y. _____

z. _____

Forgiveness Lists

How many people do you know who hold grudges? Typically, a grudge is held as if it were a precious gem. We hang onto it tightly and guard it with ferocity. Holding onto strong feelings of anger and resentment towards others is harmful. It is like holding onto a poison which gradually saps us of health and power. Harboring resentment over long periods of time, especially if we don't acknowledge it, is often a major factor that perpetuates the vicious cycle of Mind Body Syndrome. Often there is nothing we can do about the situations that bother us. If there is no direct action we can take to resolve the situation, we are left with emotional pains that serve to exacerbate physical pain.

The only way out of this condition is forgiveness. Forgiveness is a gift that you give to yourself. It is an act which allows you to free yourself from the prison of toxic emotions. Learning to forgive means that you are letting go of the emotional pain you harbor and that you choose to stop allowing a situation from the past to harm you today. It doesn't mean that the other person was "right." It means you are taking steps to free yourself and prevent another person from controlling your reactions any longer.

Most people think of forgiveness in a spiritual sense, being kind to the person who hurt you. This is a very healthy thing to do if you can. In a good relationship, it can be relatively easy to forgive a friend or sibling, especially if they apologize. It is healthy as long as we are able to let go of the emotions that were activated.

But when someone has been hurt significantly, this kind of forgiveness is often not possible. People who have been physically or sexually abused may harbor tremendous anger towards their offender. As demonstrated in the EAET techniques of emotional work, there are healthy and powerful ways of releasing this anger to heal and let go of the hurts. This is healthy as you become able to disallow that person or their actions to continue to have any control over you. It is an act of power and self-preservation to live your life by letting go of fear, resentment, and guilt.

A wonderful therapist that I work with testifies about the power of doing this work to recover from traumatic events, let go of the past, and become whole again. When Heidi was a sophomore in college, she was at a fraternity party and was date raped. For several years, she was ashamed, felt that it was her fault, and told no one. She tried to move on with her life and push it to the back of her mind, but the emotional pain remained. After college, she began to have pain in her feet and anxiety. A podiatrist diagnosed her as having neuromas in her feet and operated on one foot, removing a benign tumor of nerve tissue. The pain in that foot went away. After working with a therapist doing body-centered work similar to the MBS process, she began to express her anger at her rapist. In a metaphoric sense, she had turned that anger against her feet for not kicking him or running away. Her anxiety decreased, and the pain in her other foot went away without surgery. She took self-defense classes and earned honors in jujitsu and judo, gaining confidence. She used the trauma as a springboard to improve her life in a process known as "post-traumatic growth." At her college reunion, the man who had raped her walked up to her and asked, "Hey, remember me?" She told him no and walked away.

When you decide to forgive or express and release feelings about someone or some entity, you are taking a powerful step towards your health and towards eliminating your pain. It is that simple and that important. I have seen many people who harbor anger towards someone who injured them, often in a car accident. Since the accident occurred many months or years ago, the body tissues have healed. What is causing their current pain is that the emotional wounds have not healed. And that is something they can control!

Forgiving ourselves is necessary where we harbor guilt over something we did or didn't do. As you now know, MBS frequently develops in those of us who are self-critical and who tend to feel guilty. I treated a woman who harbored deep guilt that stemmed from her daughter's violent death.

She clung to the belief that she should have protected her daughter, despite the fact that this would have been impossible. Her pain was a way of punishing herself. Guilt is an extremely powerful emotion that is at the core of MBS in a large proportion of my patients. That is why forgiving yourself is a critical component of this program. You deserve forgiveness from yourself and from others. There are several scientific (McCullough, et. al., 2001) and general interest books (Enright, 2001; Luskin, 2002) that you can read for more information on forgiveness.

Make a list of the people that you would like to forgive for something they might have done. List people that you would like to ask for forgiveness for something you may have done. Finally, list those things for which you would like to forgive yourself.

Those you would like to forgive or release feelings towards:

a. _____

b. _____

c. _____

d. _____

e. _____

f. _____

g. _____

h. _____

i. _____

j. _____

k. _____

l. _____

m. _____

n. _____

o. _____

p. _____

q. _____

r. _____

s. _____

t. _____

u. _____

v. _____

w. _____

x. _____

y. _____

z. _____

Those you would like to ask for forgiveness:

a. _____

b. _____

c. _____

d. _____

e. _____

f. _____

g. _____

h. _____

i. _____

j. _____

k. _____

l. _____

m. _____

n. _____

o. _____

p. _____

q. _____

r. _____

Things for which you would like to forgive yourself:

a. _____

b. _____

c. _____

d. _____

e. _____

f. _____

g. _____

h. _____

i. _____

j. _____

k. _____

l. _____

m._____

n. _____

o. _____

p. _____

q. _____

r. _____

List of barriers to getting better

A common barrier to curing MBS is the way that the mind can adapt to being in pain for a long time. The pain can become part of our identity. And in a weird way, it becomes comfortable. The subconscious mind is so powerful that it can create a virtual prison for us. No one wants to be in pain. Yet there are often subconscious forces that create strong barriers to getting better.

I treated a woman who had severe pain for many years and when she started the course, her pain started to decrease. As soon as this happened, she began to feel anxious and had trouble sleeping. These are very common reactions that Freud termed symptom substitutions, situations where the mind will substitute new symptoms for old ones because it's not ready to give up having symptoms yet. It is also caused by the progress that one is making, because the mind is starting to give up the usual (old) symptoms. This woman came to the class in tears, crying these words: "I can't stand the anxiety and the sleeplessness. Give me my pain back! I'm at least used to my pain."

The subconscious mind can hang onto symptoms because these symptoms can help us avoid certain situations or get some things that we may need. If we maintain our symptoms, we may avoid having to work, to attend family functions, or fulfill certain social obligations. Some of these situations may cause us anger, fear, or anxiety. If we hang onto our symptoms, we may obtain sympathy or attention, or we may feel that we are very strong or a martyr. These are very common human reactions to life situations and to chronic symptoms. If we are brave enough and honest enough to look for these issues, we can begin to free ourselves of barriers that prevent us from getting better.

It takes a great deal of insight and courage to do this. I recall a woman who had the courage to state that she wasn't sure her husband would pay attention to her if she didn't have MBS symptoms. One man told me that a barrier for him was that if he did get better, it would mean that he actually could have gotten better several years earlier.

In the movie, *The Shawshank Redemption*, prisoners subjected to vicious and inhumane treatment when they enter prison learn to adapt to life inside the prison walls. Although consciously all of them proclaim their innocence and cannot wait to be set free, they are subconsciously affected by their physical prison and they gradually create a prison of their own within their minds. The film calls this "institutionalization," and the characters deal with this powerful force in different ways.

People are too often subjected to a process that can be termed "medicalization." Their experiences of symptoms and many unsuccessful attempts to treat it can lead to a life where the only constant is their symptoms.

Make a list of possible reasons why your mind might want to hang on to any MBS symptoms. Include things such as not having to work, not having to help with chores or family obligations, getting calls or sympathy from friends or family proving that there is a significant injury, involved in a lawsuit, etc. Do not be afraid that this list will harm you in any way. It is to uncover hidden reasons in the subconscious mind that might get in the way of ridding yourself of MBS symptoms. Everyone is likely to have some hidden barriers.

List of barriers:

a. _____

b. _____

c. _____

d. _____

e. _____

f. _____

g. _____

h. _____

i. _____

j. _____

k. _____

l. _____

m. _____

n. _____

o. _____

p. _____

q. _____

r. _____

Writing Exercises: Gratitude, Forgiveness, Barriers

Choose topics that you think are important to you or that will help you get better from the gratitude, forgiveness, and barrier lists, and write them on the corresponding lines below.

Gratitude List Topics:

1. _____

2. _____

3. _____

Forgiveness List Topics:

1. _____

2. _____

3. _____

Barriers List Topics:

1. _____

2. _____

3. _____

Each day choose one of these topics and do a free-write exercise with the instructions on the following pages. There are pages for two fast writes for each category. Do as many as necessary from each of these categories on separate paper.

Gratefulness Free-Write No. 1

I am grateful for _____ and this is why:

Gratefulness Free-Write No. 2

I am grateful for _____ and this is why:

Forgiveness Free-Write No. 1

I forgive _____ for _____ and this is why:

     OR

I ask forgiveness from _____ for _____ and this is why:

     OR

I forgive myself for _____ and this is why:

Forgiveness Free-Write No. 2

I forgive _____ for _____ and this is why:

    OR

I ask forgiveness from _____ for _____ and this is why:

    OR

I forgive myself for _____ and this is why:

Barriers Free-Write No. 1

My mind may prefer to hang on to my symptoms because _____
_____

but this is why I choose to get better and this is how I'm going to overcome this barrier:

Barriers Free-Write No. 2

My mind may prefer to hang on to my symptoms because _____

_____

but this is why I choose to get better and this is how I'm going to overcome this barrier:

Exercise: Being Open to and Accepting of Yourself

Think for several moments about what you notice about yourself. Focus on the times when you are open, accepting, and kind to yourself—those times when the "eagle" is dominant. What do you notice when you are kind, open, and accepting of yourself? How do you feel at these times? How do you act towards yourself and others? On the lines below, write down anything that comes to mind in response to these questions. Examples might be "I feel happy" or "I notice calmness." Be patient, and see what thoughts arise. List as many items as you can.

_____

_____

_____

_____

_____

_____

_____

_____

_____

_____

_____

_____

_____

The way that you feel when you are open and accepting of yourself is entirely dependent on how you look at yourself. What would it be like to spend a day (or every day) filled with the feelings you listed above? Who controls if you feel open and accepting of yourself? You do. If you'd like to spend more time feeling like your list above, all you have to do is this: When you wake up each morning, make a decision to be open and accepting of yourself that day. Allow that concept to sink into your heart and mind every day. Feel some of the feelings that you listed above each morning and remind yourself of them throughout the day. Over time, it will tend to become the way you experience yourself and your life.

The relationship between self-love and acceptance is powerfully illustrated in the following quote from a woman who is participating in this program.

"I am grateful for family and friends and the BEST CHRISTMAS EVER! I don't think I've ever enjoyed the holidays as much as I have this year. It has just been an awesome experience, every step of the way. To be able to walk and be outside in the fresh air. To be able to sit and enjoy a cup of coffee with my friends. To no longer be afraid of coffee and caffeine as a potential trigger. To be able to do my hair and dance and use the computer and read and write and cook and smile. It's just so nice to be able to live again. But the most important thing I think this Christmas is not just that I'm able to get out of bed. It's that I think for the first time in my life that I genuinely like myself. And I feel much more comfortable in my own skin. Not that I still don't have a long ways to go. But I'm getting there."

Now that you can see some of the positive characteristics that you already have within you, consider what other characteristics you would like to emphasize. You can also think about how you might be able to use some of these positive characteristics when you are faced with certain stressful situations. For example, how would you like to respond to a stressful conversation with a parent, child, sibling, friend, boss, or coworker? How would you like to respond to a frustration that arises? How would you like to respond to a flare-up of pain or other symptom?

List the characteristics that you would like to emphasize in your life:

(Examples might include being more kind to yourself, more outgoing, calmer, happier, more assertive, or worrying less)

_____

_____

_____

_____

_____

_____

_____

_____

_____

_____

_____

_____

_____

Now make a list of stressful situations that you are probably going to encounter—including those you expect to occur in the next several weeks or months.

List of situations that are likely to be stressful: (Examples might include certain conversations, meetings, frustrations, symptoms)

_____

_____

_____

_____

_____

_____

_____

_____

_____

_____

_____

_____

_____

_____

_____

_____

_____

Writing Exercise: The New You Responds

From the lists you have just created, choose a situation that is likely to be challenging to you in some way, and write about it. You can write from the point of view of the new you—how you will be, how you will act, how you will respond to certain situations in your life. The object of this exercise is to write about your role in the situation, controlling what you can as you imagine it. You can't control how others act, so don't imagine doing so; simply visualize how you will act. David Burns (1999) has written a guide for dealing with stressful situations by controlling what you can control and accepting that you can alter only your own behavior. Of course, the Serenity Prayer states that beautifully (Sifton, 2005). Incorporate the characteristics you would like to emphasize in yourself, and write about how you will think and act to "feed" these characteristics. Review the emotional worksheets that you have completed earlier. The "lessons learned" and "actions to be taken" lines can be used as a guide to how you will choose to act in these situations. Do as many of these exercises as necessary to help you plan your responses. Then incorporate these responses into your life. Complete one of these exercises each day or every other day this week. Use extra paper if necessary.

The New You Responds No.1

_____ has just happened (or will happen soon). How will you respond? What characteristics will you bring to this situation? Write the story of this situation as you'd like it to play out with the new you as the prime actor.

The New You Responds No.2

_____ has just happened (or will happen soon).

How will you respond? What characteristics will you bring to this situation? Write the story of this

situation as you'd like it to play out with the new you as the prime actor.

The New You Responds No.3

_____ has just happened (or will happen soon).

How will you respond? What characteristics will you bring to this situation? Write the story of this

situation as you'd like it to play out with the new you as the prime actor.

The New You Responds No.4

_____ has just happened (or will happen soon).

How will you respond? What characteristics will you bring to this situation? Write the story of this

situation as you'd like it to play out with the new you as the prime actor.

The New You Responds No.5

_____ has just happened (or will happen soon).

How will you respond? What characteristics will you bring to this situation? Write the story of this

situation as you'd like it to play out with the new you as the prime actor.

Meditation for Week Four: The New You

Listen to this meditation, and take time to visualize each of the images. Several studies have demonstrated that visualization can have powerful effects on physical activities (Ross, et. al., 2003; Lacourse, et. al., 2005), overall health (Trakhtenberg, 2008), and pain (MacIver, et. al., 2008).

Meditation Synopsis

Take a few moments to place yourself in a comfortable situation where you won't be disturbed. Thank yourself for taking time for yourself and for doing this important work. Breathe deeply and allow yourself to relax. Observe your breath filling your lungs completely and watch as your lungs empty fully.

Picture the times when you are open and accepting of your self. Take a few moments and let these thoughts and feelings sink in. Ask yourself: "What do I notice when I am open and accepting of myself?" Pay close attention to these thoughts and these feelings as you answer this question.

Picture yourself going through a day being open and accepting of yourself. Picture how you would feel, how you would react to others, how you would react to events and situations.

Now take a few moments to consider some of the traits and characteristics that you would like to develop in yourself. Ask yourself these questions: "What characteristics would I like to have? What kind of person would I like to be?" Take some time to answer these questions, and let the answers sink into your mind.

Next, create an image of yourself doing something that you would like to do or that you have to do. Picture yourself as you make preparations for this and as you begin to do it. Make the images as vivid and real as you can.

Picture yourself doing this activity without any pain or dysfunction. Picture yourself completing this activity or task easily and effortlessly. See this clearly, and feel yourself as you would like to be.

Picture yourself as being the way you'd like to be throughout the day—how you feel, what you do, how you respond to people, situations, and events. What kinds of things would you do?

What kinds of things would you say? Create these actions and conversations in your mind.

Finally, take a few moments to think about things you would like to do in the future. Picture yourself overcoming any barriers to doing them. Picture yourself being healthier, stronger, and more able to do these things. Picture the new you as being happier, kinder, and more loving and forgiving to yourself and to others. Picture yourself being grateful for the things you have in your life.

End this session with these wishes for yourself:

"May I be peaceful and contented,

May I be free from harm and illness,

May I be loving and loved,

May I be forgiving and forgiven."

Repeat these wishes three times.

Think of others in your life who might benefit from these wishes or others to whom you would like to send these wishes. Repeat these wishes for these people three times.

"May they be peaceful and contented,

May they be free from harm and illness,

May they be loving and loved,

May they be forgiving and forgiven."

Reprogramming the Brain: Pain Reprocessing continued

This workbook has presented a variety of methods for reprogramming the brain. They are all ways of separating yourself from pain, anxiety, depression, or other symptoms of MBS. You have learned to separate from the symptoms by being assertive and taking control over them, by using affirmations to change neural programming in the brain and body, by activating new pathways connecting the body to the brain (such as with acupuncture points or by havening techniques), and by laughing at the symptoms to demonstrate they have no power over you. This week, we present a very powerful method of separating from the painful symptoms by meeting them without flinching and accepting they are tolerable and transient. It requires a deep sense of peace within yourself to observe the painful sensations while knowing you are OK.

This level of mindfulness allows you to relax even in the presence of physical or emotional pain. It takes time and practice to learn this method, which helps deal with the inevitable ups and downs of life. When pain, fear or other symptoms arise, practice just sitting with them. Observe them and allow your mind to engage with them without fear. Label them as "sensations" rather than as pain, anxiety or other symptoms. This is very important and will help you shift away from your symptoms. Notice whether they change as you pay attention to them; they will likely seem worse or better. Don't worry, but just return your mind to observing without fear. One of my patients said that this is like being a Jedi Master, staring down the pain or the anxiety. It takes courage, but do it with complete knowledge that you are not broken, and with strong compassion and kindness for yourself and with knowing that you will get better, and you will find this a powerful way to overcome MBS. You can practice this as a meditative exercise by going to unlearnyourpain.com, clicking on the Unlearn Your Pain Meditations, using the password: meditations, and choosing the Mindful Awareness Exercise.

We have the capacity to alter how we interpret a variety of sensations that we experience. For example, few people enjoy the taste of spicy foods, beer or whiskey initially. However, many of us train ourselves to like these tastes over time. Similarly, many people learn to enjoy the feeling of muscle discomfort that occurs with strenuous exercise. I have found that it is possible at times for my patients to interpret their physical sensations as less unpleasant or neutral, rather than as painful and uncomfortable. Obviously, severe pain is unlikely ever to be pleasant, but some sensations such as tingling, numbness, or fullness can be viewed during a mindful awareness exercise as being not as unpleasant or even slightly pleasant. This helps to detach from it and worry less about it, which in turn, decreases the danger signal.

There is another technique where you can "play" with the symptoms. For example, you can imagine turning the symptom into a certain favorite color or putting sparkles on it. One patient had abdominal pain that seemed to run in a horizontal fashion over her upper abdomen. While doing a mindful awareness exercise, she noted that it had shifted to vertical. I asked if she could ask her brain to shift it again into a diagonal orientation and it did! She was amazed and gained further proof that this was her brain and that the symptoms could and would change. When you do this, you are reversing the fear associated with your symptoms and taking strides towards freedom.

Here is another method for reversing fear and reducing pain. A recent research study showed that people who are able to tolerate and express a wide variety of feelings are better adjusted and healthier (Quoidbach, et. al., 2014). As you sit in meditation and as you go through your day, pay attention to feelings that arise, such as annoyance, anger, frustration, anxiety, fear, sadness, and pain. Allow yourself to feel them fully, knowing that they are transient, then observe them and detach from them and watch them pass on. Meet yourself and your day with kindness, love, and gratefulness for simply being alive and being able to give to yourself and others.

As you let negative feelings go, focus on letting go of self-blame and lack of self-worth. You are a living being on this earth, and you deserve to be here, to be full of life, and to be grateful for what you have. Stop focusing on the pain, and focus on loving yourself and loving others. Accept your whole self, all of your goodness and all of your flaws. Practice accepting others in this same fashion. Be grateful for the ups and the downs that life has given you, the opportunities to learn from and the obstacles to overcome. Make amends to yourself and forgive yourself for your flaws, just as you would forgive someone you love dearly. Practice forgiving others for their flaws. Separate from pain as you act to be a force for goodness in the world. Believe that you can change your life and your pain. You have the power to change the negative programming of your past and move forward. The more you focus on your purpose, the more you let go of your painful past. The more you focus on positive relationships, the more you let go of your fears and pain.

People who have a sense of purpose and meaning in their lives and who develop strong connections with other people are happier and have less pain and illness. Practice being loving, accepting, and grateful on a regular basis. It is not always easy, but it is a powerful method of healing. It may seem impossible at times, but as you work at it, you will find that gradually you will be able to replace pain, anxiety, and depression with peacefulness and wisdom. As you expand your view of the world to focus less on your daily issues and pay more attention to your place in the world and your ability to connect to others and help others, you will be more at peace with yourself, and your mind and body will let go of tension that perpetuates pain.

If you are having trouble feeling compassion towards yourself, practice feeling compassion towards someone or something. Picture a child or close friend or relative or an animal or even someone in the news. Encourage yourself to feel kindness and send out compassion to that person or animal. Then extend that same compassion to yourself as a child or when you were under stress. Look at yourself in the mirror with kindness.

When pain, anxiety, or depression arises, you can meet those feelings with love rather than resistance. You can thank the symptoms for alerting you to problems. Like a smoke alarm, they served their purpose. You can send kind and caring messages, send feelings of compassion to your symptom. You can send love to your head or neck or leg. You can give kindness to the danger signal in your brain to calm it and soothe it, just as you would calm and soothe a child who has hurt herself or is afraid of a thunderstorm. Calm and soothe yourself as well.

Another way to leave pain behind is to focus on positive things in your life and connect your brain and its neural pathways to them. The more you do that, the more you are training your brain to activate positive pathways. Try this exercise: Think back to a time in your life when you were feeling happy, peaceful, joyous, free, or in awe. Close your eyes and imagine that you are now in that time. Allow yourself to feel the positive feelings you felt then. Breathe in these positive feelings deeply and let them spread into your heart and brain and all of your body. Accept that negative feelings will arise as well, but allow them to pass so you can go back to feeling contentment. If you notice internal voices of criticism, don't linger on them, but let them pass as well and return your mind to the time when you were feeling free and comfortable. Let your mind stay with these positive feelings for as long as you want. As those feelings spread through your body, recognize they can be present in your everyday life. You can learn to access these feelings on a more regular basis as you practice noticing them. You can take moments during your day to go to these feelings. You can look for moments that are interesting, curious, happy, or peaceful and take time to allow those feelings to flourish.

Finally, you can look for things to do that will help you access these feelings. You can visit people who you enjoy. You can watch or listen to enjoyable movies or TV shows. You can dance or sing. You can practice being kind to yourself and to others. The more you take time for positive things, the more time your brain is healing rather than suffering.

We all have some stressful situations and difficult times. And we also have positive things in our lives. When we practice meeting the good and the bad with peacefulness, serenity, kindness, gratefulness, and love, we are nurturing attitudes that lead to recovery from MBS.

For many people, the learned neural pathways of pain and other symptoms have been present for a long time. In addition, the personality traits that have contributed to MBS are likely to have been present even longer. These personality traits include putting themselves last, of neglecting their own needs, of being self-critical, and of not caring for themselves or not standing up for themselves. Since these are also learned neural pathways, it is often crucial to reverse them in order to recover.

Since your brain is sending you messages almost constantly that you're damaged or broken, that you are not worthy, and that you are in danger, you will need to counteract these messages. Use this exercise on a regular basis.

Take time each day to stop and remind yourself that you are well, you are healthy, you are strong, you are not damaged, and that you are safe. Tell yourself that you are a good person, that you are important, that you "count" and that you "matter." Send messages of kindness and caring and love to yourself. Do this over and over again. Believe these messages, because they are the truth. The part of your brain that is trying to scare you will gradually relax as these truths sink in. This may take some time, but you will succeed as you allow yourself to let go of the false messages that your brain has been sending and gradually change these personality traits. This is the long and difficult work of altering your relationship with yourself. It is probably the most important work you will do. Don't despair, and don't give up. You hold the key to your recovery.

It is almost impossible to explain how important self-compassion is in recovery from MBS. Emotional hurts are compounded by self-neglect, which is one of the most important components in the development of MBS. Vicky wrote this about her healing journey:

"Lucky. That's how at 18 years old, I described being raped at knifepoint by an intruder in my very first apartment. Lucky. A lot of women get raped and murdered, I told myself. I'm still alive, so I have no right to feel sorry for myself, to be angry. Thirty years later, debilitating migraine headaches led me to read Unlearn Your Pain. I got angry at my rapist for the very first time. I screamed, "You have no right to touch me!" over and over until decades of pain erupted like an exploding volcano. I imagined my neighbor and I kicking his crumbling ass to the ground in the narrow courtyard of the apartment building. I finished the story with the police arresting him. I began to heal a wound I never even knew I had.

I don't remember ever thinking I deserved to feel compassion for myself, no matter how bad the situation. There was always someone who had it worse than I did. This caused me to take care of everyone else and put everyone's needs before mine. This personality trait, a toxic concoction brewed from an upbringing I now think must be the most common of my generation: 60s & 70s girls reared by 50s moms. My mother loved me, something I never doubted. But I also could not reveal myself emotionally to her without having her judge me. So instead of letting things out, from very early on, I began to catalogue an extensive library of fear and shame and trauma deep in my subconscious, completely without my knowledge. Just deal with it and keep smiling. Throughout my life, this trait earned me all kinds of praise, "She's so strong…She's so nice…She can handle ANYTHING." No one ever saw me upset, or angry, or grumpy, or rude.

I did everything I could to ignore my body and brain's attempts to get my attention. It wasn't just chronic migraines. My back went into spasms during a bad marriage. I doubled over in abdominal pain for 9 months under the subordination of a terrible boss. The day I was set to start my field work for my master's of geology, traversing a 14-thousand-foot volcano alone, both my knees collapsed beneath me. I just kept going but never connected the dots; never understood what these symptoms signified.

That is, until three months of crippling pain forced me to dissect my very soul. What I found was that the person in my life who was doing me the most harm, the person who held the key to my chronic pain and the only one who could unlock the mystery of my anguish, was me. The realization of how much pain I had caused myself now layered upon me a heavy blanket of sadness and grief. To heal, I needed to allow myself to feel; to feel the grief as it welled up and flowed out of me, and to feel the anger. Not only did I have anger towards the rapist, but towards my own mother; and to someone else. I found that I would literally have to divide myself in half. On one side, I would have to express anger toward A PART OF ME—for 40 years of utter neglect of my emotional needs. This anger came quickly, boiled up unexpectedly, and gave me an instant feeling of healing from physical symptoms in my chest and head.

My migraines have all but subsided. Healing the other part of me is more difficult and ultimately more important. It is the painstaking process of rebuilding a broken relationship. It is the reconnecting with someone I abandoned long ago. And it is the learning—maybe for the first time—to be a loving and compassionate caretaker of myself."

Dealing with Difficult Situations

You are probably aware of some issues or situations that are unfinished and still bother you. These may involve business situations where money is owed or relationships where feelings were hurt. Conflicts often occur between people which are left unresolved for many years.

Make a list of things that you need to do, finish, resolve, or take care of. On this list, place anything that still weighs on your mind, even if you're not sure you can do anything to resolve it, and even if doing something about it would be very difficult or even impossible.

In one of my classes, there was a married woman who was diagnosed with fibromyalgia and had a tremendous amount of physical pain. A major stressor was that her sister-in-law was spreading false rumors that she was having an affair. When she came to this point in the program, she decided to confront her sister-in-law. They met, and she explained that she was not having an affair and told her to stop spreading the rumors. Within days, her pain melted away.

Sometimes we just need to act—by doing certain exercises or work, by pushing our bodies to do things we have been avoiding, by expressing ourselves to others, or by changing our work or a relationship situation in some way. If you are in a situation or relationship that continues to be hurtful to you, you need to protect yourself. Make important decisions carefully, but it is sometimes necessary to alter or end certain business or social relationships. Standing up for oneself is often the key to ending a painful relationship and the beginning of healing MBS.

Make a list of:

Things that you need to do,

Things that you should take care of,

Things that are important for you to resolve (even if they may be difficult)

_____

_____

_____

_____

_____

_____

_____

_____

_____

_____

_____

_____

_____

_____

_____

_____

_____

_____

_____

_____

_____

_____

_____

Choose two or three items from this list and decide what you might be able to do about them. At this time, you might only be able to do a free-write on the subject to begin to recognize your feelings. Or you just may be able to write an unsent letter. You might be able to write a letter and send it or call the person involved and discuss the issue. You might be able to meet with the person and apologize or ask for forgiveness. You might need to ask someone to do something that needs to be done. You may need to make up your mind and take action.

Write one item from your list on this line _____

Consider what you could do about this in the next week or two. Write those options on the following lines.

_____

_____

_____

_____

_____

_____

_____

_____

_____

_____

_____

Choose an initial plan of action. Write it here.

_____

_____

_____

_____

_____

Set a deadline for accomplishing this task in the next week or two.

Figure out how you're going to accomplish this task. Who can help you? Who can you ask for advice? Can someone go with you? How are you going to accomplish the task? What barriers might occur, and how will you overcome them?

Write a paragraph answering these questions.

Make a commitment to this task. Even though these tasks may be very difficult, most people feel much better after they accomplish them. Even if your first step is a small one, it will often give you the courage and confidence to take a slightly larger step if the issue is still unresolved.

After you have accomplished your task, write a brief paragraph describing what happened, how you felt, and what this accomplished.

Now that you've accomplished one small task on this issue, was this enough to help you resolve or finish this issue? Do you need to take a further step? Or can you move on to another issue that needs to be resolved?

Consider what this next step might be and go through the same process as you did before. Remember that while taking these steps can be difficult, the results are almost always positive and you will feel better both emotionally and physically when you have been able to complete these tasks.

Choose another issue that needs resolving, and write that item from your list on this line.

_____

Consider what you could do about this in the next week or two. Write those options on the following lines.

_____

_____

_____

_____

_____

_____

_____

_____

_____

_____

Choose an initial plan of action. Write it here.

_____

_____

_____

_____

_____

_____

Set a deadline for accomplishing this task in the next week or two.

_____

Figure out how you're going to accomplish this task. Who can help you? Who can you ask for advice? Can someone go with you? How are you going to accomplish the task? What barriers might occur, and how will you overcome them?

Write a paragraph answering these questions.

Make a commitment to this task. Even though these tasks may be difficult, most people feel much better after they accomplish them. Even if your first step is a small one, it will often give you the courage and confidence to take a slightly larger step if the issue is still unresolved.

After you have accomplished your task, write a brief paragraph describing what happened, how you felt, and what this accomplished.

Choose another issue that needs resolving, and write that item from your list on this line.

_____

Consider what you could do about this in the next week or two. Write those options on the following lines.

_____

_____

_____

_____

_____

_____

_____

_____

Choose an initial plan of action. Write it here.

_____

_____

_____

_____

_____

_____

Set a deadline for accomplishing this task in the next week or two.

_____

Figure out how you're going to accomplish this task. Who can help you? Who can you ask for advice? Can someone go with you? How are you going to accomplish the task? What barriers might occur, and how will you overcome them?

Write a paragraph answering these questions.

Make a commitment to this task. Even though these tasks may be very difficult, most people feel much better after they accomplish them. Even if your first step is a small one, it will often give you the courage and confidence to take a slightly larger step if the issue is still unresolved.

After you have accomplished your task, write a brief paragraph describing what happened, how you felt, and what this accomplished.

Facing Fears and Choosing a New Life

Some people can become overwhelmed by fear while doing this work. Fear is the basis of MBS and the driving force in activating and perpetuating pain. Fear activates pain pathways in the brain, and pain activates fear pathways in the brain, and that interaction can lead to a vicious cycle. Some of my patients are consumed by fearful thoughts all the time and find it hard to shake them. If you are like that, here are some methods of reversing fear, freeing your mind to start to lift pain, anxiety, or depression.

If fear dominates your thinking, try this exercise. Take a piece of paper and divide it into two columns. At the top of the left column, write "Fearful thoughts," and at the top of the right column, write "Opposites." List all your fearful thoughts and the arguments against them. They might include:

I could be paralyzed	I am not paralyzed
I might die	I will live
I could kill myself	I will not kill myself
I will be in pain forever	I will recover from pain
My body is wracked with arthritis	My body is healthy and strong
I have herniated discs	Herniated discs do not cause my pain
I hate myself	I can love myself
I don't deserve to be pain free	I deserve to be pain free
My body is damaged beyond repair	My body can heal
I will never be happy	I can and will be happy

At the bottom of the page, write something like this:

I can choose what I believe; I choose not to live in fear. Fear will arise, but I can handle it, even though it's uncomfortable. As I face and tolerate fear, it makes me stronger, because I can handle it. I choose life for myself, I will not fear having fear so I can be free.

Then cut your paper in half and burn, shred, tear, or otherwise destroy the column on the left. While doing so, smile or laugh at the fearful thoughts. You can do this same exercise on your phone, tablet, or computer, erasing the fearful thoughts and saving the thoughts that affirm you as a person who can choose your destiny. See how you feel as you let go of fearful thoughts and embrace positive thoughts.

Keep the column that lists the rebuttals to your fear and refer to it when fearful thoughts arise during the day. Say to yourself with a smile: "I already did my worrying for the day. Those thoughts are in the wastebasket." Then you can reach into your pocket to touch your positive thoughts or read them in order to reconnect with them.

A man who did this exercise observed: "I think the one idea that really hit home with me is that I have a choice. It is my choice whether I am going to allow pain to control my life and my future or am I going to control my life and my future."

Some years ago, an American and a German were each in dire straits. They were depressed, overcome with fear and feelings of worthlessness. Both Byron Katie (*Loving What Is*, 2002) and Eckhart Tolle (*The Power of Now*, 1999) had an awakening. They both realized that they were telling themselves a false story, believing self-defeating thoughts as if these thoughts were true. When they challenged them, they recovered. The stories we tell ourselves have great power over us.

Both Katie and Tolle realized that they were not sick or damaged and that their negative thoughts were an illusion, not the truth. Doctors have told many of my patients that they were damaged in some ways and that they would never recover. Sometimes even support groups are filled with people who do not believe in the possibility of recovery. But you do not have to believe the lie that you are irreparably damaged. You can choose to believe that you have the power to recover.

William James, the father of modern psychology, was a brilliant and innovative thinker. However, when he was growing up in the mid-1800s, he was troubled by many ailments, including abdominal and back pains and severe depression. He contemplated suicide many times. However, before taking such drastic action, he did an experiment. He decided to tell himself each morning that he believed that he could change (Duhigg, 2012). He did this for a year, and this simple act changed his outlook and his life.

A good first step in dealing with fear is to assess it for its validity. Are you really in significant danger right now? Must you believe that you are damaged or in danger? Look more deeply at your life and your body and discard the illusion. In truth you are healthy, not diseased, and you have the ability to recover from your pain, anxiety, or depression. Begin to move past fearful thoughts.

As Tolle and many others have discovered, mindfulness meditation techniques can conquer fear. You are not your thoughts. Thoughts are mental constructs. Everyone at times has scary thoughts, even thoughts of harming themselves or others, and these fearful thoughts are part of the danger/alarm mechanism. They are trying to scare you and pull you back into fear. You can choose to observe them, rather than believe or fear them. Such thoughts are normal. Listen to the meditation entitled Mindfulness Meditation from chapter 7 at unlearnyourpain.com, Meditations tab, password: meditations. Practice simply noticing all your thoughts as they arise. They are "just thoughts" that will go away if you simply notice them, separate from them, and watch them as they come and go and your mind replaces them with other thoughts and focuses on other things.

But fear doesn't just reside in the mind. It also lives in our bodies. Notice fear in how your body reacts to life events. You can begin to alter these sensations of fear by moving your body through them. When you begin to feel fear in your body, tell your brain that you know it is producing these sensations and that they are not harmful or dangerous. Then try doing something active, such as exercises, fast walking, or dancing. Take that fearful energy and use it in a positive way.

A mindful approach to dealing with fearful sensations in the body is to simply sit and observe them, allowing yourself to be with them without judging them or fearing them. Separate from them; feel them without reacting to them. If you do not resist them, they will decrease and go away. If you like, visualize them in some way and then use a visual image to calm them or wash them away. Finally, you can encourage yourself to feel them fully as a way of challenging yourself to be with them without being afraid of them. By doing this, you can prove to yourself you can tolerate these thoughts. You can practice this by using a guided meditation on my website. Go to unlearnyourpain.com, click on the Meditations tab, use the password: meditations and choose the Embracing Emotions meditation.

Once you have the understanding that you have MBS and you express your deepest feelings, the addition of mindfulness practice can have powerful effects. At her initial appointment with me, Erin was sure that she had MBS and I helped her to recognize and express some anger that was at the core of her symptoms. However, she wasn't immediately better and she wrote this a few days later.

AFTER READING Unlearn Your Pain *and having an appointment with Dr. Schubiner, I now knew that I had MBS, and I expected to be cured quickly. However, when I still had so much pain, I became frustrated and hopeless. I had three really rough days of despair and pain, filled with tears and anger. And then something shifted. I was reading The Power of Now and something clicked for me: I realized that I had to take care of myself; no one was going to do it or me. Even though I was trapped in an endless obsession of thoughts, fears and pain,*

I was responsible for it at some deep level. Then I started to focus on my breath and worked on letting everything else go. There, I found comfort and caring for myself and I could imagine that I would not always be suffering. I began to separate from the pain and even though I still had pain, it was just a sensation. I began to develop a sense of empowerment and began to let go of fear. And then pain disappeared, and even though it came back later, I wasn't as obsessed with it or worried about it. I now know that I am on the right path and no matter how long it takes I will be OK. I held the key all along, yet I never realized it. I am seeing the pain gradually recede as I let go of fear.

If You Are Not Yet Improving

At this point in the program, some people begin to wonder if this approach will work for them, especially if they have not begun to see results. Although changes in pain can occur very quickly, there are also many people who don't experience these changes for a couple of weeks, or even longer. If you have any concerns about the program at this point, please read the following.

1. Erase doubt.

Recognize that your true diagnosis is MBS and that the symptoms you are experiencing are completely due to the interaction between the mind and the body. If you begin to doubt if you truly have MBS or you begin to wonder if some other purely physical condition is present, you will be undermining your recovery by creating a subconscious barrier, as described in this chapter. Contact your doctor if you think some new physical condition has developed, but be aware that symptoms of MBS typically shift and move around when you start doing this work. If you are going to succeed in this program, it is essential to maintain an unwavering commitment to the understanding that your diagnosis is MBS and that by working in this way, you will succeed in getting rid of your symptoms. Recognize that it is very common to have some difficulties in truly believing that your condition is caused by your brain. There is a tremendous drive to believe that there is some kind of tissue damage. Every time pain rises up, fear is activated, and many people get thrown right back into despair. It's as if there is a battle going on inside your brain. My colleague, Alan Gordon, of the Pain Psychology Center in Los Angeles, uses this analogy. The battle going on is like a trial in your brain, and there are two lawyers and a judge. One lawyer is using scare tactics and spreading fear. This lawyer is very experienced and uses every trick in the book to persuade you of his case. However, his client is guilty (of creating MBS symptoms in you), and he distorts the facts to convince you of his lies. His tactic is simply to scare you with FEAR, which in this case stands for False Evidence Appearing Real. On the other hand, there is a young lawyer with less experience; however, she is sincere, smart, and tells the truth. She knows that the client is guilty and has all of the facts on her side. You are the judge in this case. You must decide who is telling the truth. Examine the case thoroughly; don't be fooled by lies; don't fall for tricks and false evidence appearing real. The truth will set you free.

2. Be patient.

Your symptoms have probably been present for a fairly long time. They may take some time to go away. Don't worry if you aren't seeing immediate results. If you keep working on the program, you will begin to see results. Don't try too hard, and don't get more stressed by worrying about doing the program perfectly. As long as you know that you have MBS and also have the confidence that you will get better, you will be fine. Most patients I have seen would be relatively happy to know that they will get better, even if it takes several months. In fact, putting a time frame on your recovery can get in the way. This can be a tricky situation. You obviously want your MBS symptoms to go away. But the more you want them to go away and the more that you "can't stand them," the message you are inadvertently giving to your brain is this: "I can't take it anymore. I'm afraid of these symptoms. I don't know if they will ever go away." These, of course, are fearful thoughts and worries, which is exactly the response that the danger signal is trying to create in you. It is this attitude that further activates the danger signal to continue this vicious cycle of pain-fear-pain. So, it is critical to see this and avoid trying too hard, avoid putting time pressure on yourself to get better, and avoid fighting your symptoms. Know that you will get better and that you can't put a time table on when that happens. You just need to stay calm and patient and persist, even though that can be difficult. This twenty-eight-day program is enough for many but not all people. Use this program as a starting point for your healing journey, and you will be in a very good position to get better.

3. Keep working.

Continue to keep working on the program. Don't give up. Many people tend to avoid doing the homework, don't find the time, or procrastinate about it. This is another way that your mind can create barriers to recovery. Trust in this program, and trust in yourself. Choose the issues you think you need to work on, and use the writing and the meditations to deal with them. Make sure you do the reprogramming the brain exercises, and don't forget to take time for yourself.

4. Expect some up and downs.

There are a few people who have relatively quick and dramatic results from this program. But unfortunately, these people are in the minority. The recovery stories that are often told, including in this book, are often these. But it is much more common that it takes time to recover and that the path to recovery has ups and downs along the way. The brain's danger signal has been turned on, in some people for much of their lives. It will never turn off completely as we need it to alert us to dangers, such as acute injuries and stressful situations. It is there to protect us. However, when it's alerting us by causing pain when we are not injured, we need to turn it down! In order to do this, we need to send it consistent messages of safety over time. And the danger signal will turn down, but usually it also has times when it flares up again. Most people can expect this so that pain or other MBS symptoms will rise again. Don't be discouraged or frustrated or upset by this; it is part of the recovery process. When your symptoms go down, you can be happy. But when they return, you should also try to be happy (that may be hard!), as this will give you the opportunity to remain calm and understanding in the face of symptoms. When you do that, you are sending a powerful message to your brain that you are NOT in danger and this message works to reprogram the brain out of MBS.

5. Know thyself.

Be willing to look at your life and the things that have happened. Be willing to be honest with yourself. Everyone has done things they wish they hadn't or things they are ashamed of. Everyone has had things happen to them that they wish had never happened. It will help to recall these things and deal with them through the writing and meditating exercises. The more you are able to be honest with yourself and be kind to yourself, the more you will be able to accept yourself and let go of some of the stressful emotions that cause MBS symptoms. Practice being honest and kind with others as well.

6. Find inner strength.

Most people have had times in their lives when they made good decisions, stood up for themselves, and acted to protect themselves. In order to recover from MBS, most people need to find the inner strength to stop fearing the symptoms and take control over them. It is often helpful to look back at your life to identify the times when you have acted decisively on your own behalf. If you have done this in the past, you can do it now. It takes courage to reverse MBS. Dig deep within yourself. Day by day, find the strength to keep going and to work through any emotional issues and life situations that come your way.

7. Find contentment.

Find ways to be content or happy. Find things to be grateful for. Do things that you like and that give you pleasure. Find ways to relax. Do things for others that will give you happiness. Seek help from friends, family, co-workers, and counselors to gain support and understanding. Listen to others, and see if they will listen to you. Connecting to others in a deep way leads to an improved sense of self.

8. Do something.

Become more active. Challenge yourself physically by doing some things that you haven't done due to pain or fear. Complete your lists of activities you would like to do, and include some things that you can start doing immediately. The more active you are, the less time you will have to be in pain and the quicker you will get better.

Writing Exercise: Write Your Life Story in a New Way

Everyone has a narrative or a story they tell themselves about their lives. These stories are very powerful, not only because they remind us of our past but because they also affect our future, since to a large degree we tend to think what we can accomplish is controlled by what happened in our past. However, there are many ways to view the past and many opportunities to alter our futures. This exercise gives you the opportunity to create a new life story.

Your Old Story:

First, write a synopsis or short version of your old story: the one where you emphasize the negative things that have happened in your life and how you tend to be limited by this view of yourself. In this version, we frequently see ourselves as a victim of sorts—bad things happen to us, and we are unable to change them or rise above them. Keep this relatively short because you don't want to dwell on it.

Your New Story:

Now, write a new story for yourself. You can take the facts about things that have occurred, but try to put a new twist on them. Write about what you have learned from them and how you have (or will) overcome significant stressors or barriers. Emphasize the positive things that have happened to you and your positive reactions to life events. Emphasize your successes and things you have accomplished. This is an opportunity to view yourself as a hero—someone who has faced great odds yet finds a way to overcome them and triumph. If you can look at your life as a "hero's journey," you will be better equipped to deal with adversity and to change your life in important ways.

As you do this exercise, you will be creating the person you would like to be. Create the person who you really are: able to make new choices, able to overcome past problems, able to accomplish the things that you would like to accomplish.

Last Thoughts

This book describes in detail the negative consequences of too much stress, especially when stressful events first occur early in life and pile up later in life. When we feel overwhelmed by stress, our brains can react by producing pain, anxiety, depression, or many other MBS symptoms. These can alert us to the stress and help us to take appropriate action. This book offers a wide variety of ways to turn off the symptoms.

Stress is part of life, and we all must learn to deal with it. New research on stress points to better ways of coping with it. When we get stressed, our bodies produce hormones and chemicals to help us cope. These reactions are designed to sharpen our thinking and make our bodies ready for challenges. Research has shown that how we view stress is critical in determining how it affects us. People who feel that stress is harmful to their health are more likely to develop physical illnesses (Nabi, 2013). Individuals who are given information about the positive aspects of stress perform better under pressure (Crum, et. al., 2013). People who view their jobs as being healthy for them tend to be healthier (Crum, et. al., 2007). In fact, significant life difficulties can lead to an overall improvement in life for some people. This is called post-traumatic growth. People who use the challenges in their life positively can often make profound changes in their mind, their attitudes, and their lives. I have worked with many people with cancer and other diseases who have made positive changes in their lives because of their illness. The same is true for MBS. Although the symptoms can be severe, there is the potential for a great deal of growth during the healing process. As you reflect on your life, you will see how you can make changes, such as setting boundaries in relationships, forgiving others, or making changes in your work situation. You may also need to make internal changes like accepting yourself, treating yourself better, and being grateful for your life on a deeper level.

Here is a quote about healing and growth from a woman using the program.

"After using the Unlearn Your Pain program, my leg is feeling quite a bit better and I am learning to stop being afraid of it. But better than that, I have had severe anxiety and panic my whole life. I have not driven alone in 30 years nor do I stay at home alone. After reading your book, I was able to start facing my fears as a whole and I have started staying home alone a bit and doing many more things that I haven't been able to do in many years. People have looked at me all of my life thinking that I was afraid of everything, but I was really just afraid of the panic attacks. It was all really just about the fear. Now that I understand how the brain works, I have been able to change my life. I always wondered who

I would have been had certain things not happened to me as a child that set me on a path of anxiety. I feel like I'm finding out now."

Here's another quote from a man who is participating in this program.

"I am deeply grateful for the role that MBS has had in my life. The unique way it has impacted me. The one diamond that is forged from the fires of MBS is that it offers you an opportunity, time and time again, to finally and eventually take a stand as your own best friend. I believe that I will never in my heart of hearts betray myself again. I'm no one special, but I've earned my self-respect. There will be moments, perhaps extended periods, when I will again be bewildered, self-doubtful and confused, but I will land on my feet because I have found a home within myself and I've discovered that the instincts of my heart can be trusted.

Many examples in this book focus on people who have had fairly rapid recoveries. These true stories help you see that recovery is possible. But many others did not recover quickly. In order to succeed in this program, it is critical to believe you can recover in time, even if there are some ups and downs along the way. Studies have shown that people who are ready for improvements as well as for setbacks do better in the long run. Those who assume that everything will be easy often have trouble adjusting to setbacks. For many people, the road to the development of MBS has been long and filled with stressful life events. It can take a great deal of work to develop the necessary amounts of compassion for self and the courage to take control over the symptoms and to leave fear behind. At times, it can be a long, slow process of recovery. But don't give up. This challenging work will pay off. The gains you make will be long lasting. This work can be like breaking a difficult habit like smoking or overcoming an addiction like alcoholism. Success may require many attempts at changing thinking and behavior.

Your MBS symptoms may vary dramatically from day to day or week to week. Some people find that the symptoms get much better but then recur, or they have good days and bad days. This is very common. Some people expect that the MBS symptoms will never return. That's not usually true. I get MBS symptoms from time to time and sometimes they are quite severe. As someone who teaches others to overcome MBS, this is humbling. But I have learned that this is part of living. As someone who is prone to MBS, I realize that my mind will produce symptoms at times when I am stressed. Sometimes, I don't even know what is causing the symptom or what I am stressed about. But I tell myself, "I'm an MBS type of person, and I get MBS. I can't allow that fact to bother me or ruin my life. It's a part of my life, and the symptoms will come and they will go." Do not get upset if MBS symptoms occur in the future. Worrying about them, fearing them, and thinking that they will never go away are thoughts that tend to make MBS persist. Recognize that having some MBS symptoms at times can be a part of life, and you will be able to deal with them if they arise.

My colleague, Dr. Peter Zafirides (2013), emphasizes aspects of the human condition in his work that are known as existential, in other words, thoughts and feelings that everyone faces at some time. These include the following: 1) being separate from others, and therefore in many respects, alone; 2) making important decisions, that is, having the freedom and responsibility of choice; 3) creating meaning in our lives, that is, finding our reasons for being on this earth; and 4) facing our mortality and the inevitability of dying. At times of crisis, these issues are often important to address by recognizing them, talking and writing about them, and connecting to others, such as relatives, friends or therapists, in acknowledgment of our shared frailties and humanity.

The psychologist, Mihaly Csikszentmihalyi, described the state of "flow" in the 1970s as the feeling of being completely engaged in a task. When in the state of flow, one loses track of time due to being engrossed in the challenge of accomplishing or experiencing something meaningful. Those who are deprived of the experience of flow become irritable, distracted and have pain. One of the best ways to overcome MBS is to devote yourself to something that leads to the state of flow. This can be done through deeply engaging in work, hobbies, relationships, sports or other activities.

Another colleague of mine, Dr. David Hanscom, emphasizes the benefits of "play." When you engage in activities that are simply fun, you engage a part of your brain that turns off pain and other MBS symptoms. The book, *Play: How it Shapes the Brain, Opens the Imagination, and Invigorates the Soul,* by Stuart Brown and Vaughan (2009) describes how play alters the brain. Many adults never find time to engage in play, such as singing, dancing, drawing, sports, and laughing; and many had childhoods where they weren't encouraged to play. You may need to force yourself to find time for play, especially playful activities that have no specific purpose or value other than to enjoy the moment. For example, finger painting is a perfect playful pursuit. Regular play is one of the best ways to help people who feel stuck in physical or emotional pain.

Recent studies have shown that the two major social predictors of health and longevity are social connection (Holt-Lunstad, et. al., 2010) and meaning and purpose in life (Hill, et. al., 2014). The more you are able to emphasize and nurture strong connections to people in your life, the greater satisfaction you will have. In addition, the more you are able to identify areas of your life that give you meaning and purpose, the quicker you will recover. Who do you live for and what do you live for? Focus and act on the answers to these questions, and MBS symptoms will decrease over time.

In *Man's Search for Meaning*, Viktor Frankl describes life in a concentration camp under the Nazis. In spite of being trapped in hideous conditions, he talks of having a choice. Frankl asserts that you always have the ability to choose your attitude towards yourself and your environment. He describes finding meaning in suffering, in the hope for a better life and in maintaining loving feelings towards oneself and others. People with MBS often feel completely trapped and overwhelmed. Know that you can always choose your attitude and find purpose and meaning in your life. As you develop hope, compassion, and purpose, you will be sowing the seeds for your recovery.

chapter 11

Next Steps: Charting Your Future

Now I become myself. It's taken
Time, many years and places;
I have been dissolved and shaken,
Worn other people's faces… — May Sarton

When you get into a tight place and everything
goes against you until it seems that you cannot hold on
for a minute longer, never give up then, for that is
just the place and time when the tide will turn. — Harriet Beecher Stowe

You are now finishing the four-week program (or maybe it took a bit

longer), and you can be proud of all the hard work you've done. Hopefully, you've learned a great deal about Mind Body Syndrome and how it has impacted your life. You have probably discovered many things about yourself along the way. This program is designed not only to help you understand MBS and conquer it, but to take more control of your life and take steps toward a better future. What steps will help you improve further? Some of you have already seen great progress in reducing or eliminating your MBS symptoms. For others, you may have found only limited improvement to date. This chapter gives guidance on how to proceed in either of these situations.

For Those Yet to Complete Their Recovery

Not everyone who does this program will find relief quickly. MBS can be tricky sometimes. Our minds can find ways to thwart our progress and cling to MBS symptoms. Stay as positive as you can. Remember that the pain pathways probably developed a long time ago, and it may take a while to overcome them. It's worth another few weeks or months to get better if you know you are on the right path. For some people, it takes up to a year for their brains to be rewired and their pain to resolve. If you are having a hard time believing that you can get better, you might want to visit these two websites: www.thankyoudrsarno.com and www.tmswiki.org. The former has testimonials from people who have recovered from chronic pain by reading books by Dr. John Sarno, who taught me about this work. The latter is an excellent peer-run site for information about MBS.

One of the most important and common barriers to getting better is the persistent belief that there is something physically wrong with your body. You might think, "Maybe I really have a problem with my back from that injury," or "Maybe the doctors missed something on their exam or their testing," or "I wonder if I should get another medical opinion." If you have thoughts such as these, it is critical to deal with them quickly. To get better, you must be completely certain that your symptoms are caused by MBS—doubt can lead to fear and/or despair. If you are not sure that you have MBS, seek out doctors who can carefully review your situation, your exam, and your testing. See the lists at PPDAssociation.org, tmswiki.org, or painreprocessingtherapy.com for a doctor who has experience in MBS, or you can see a doctor in your area that you trust. (You might want to have your doctor read the first few chapters of this book.)

If you are confident that you do have MBS, you have several options. One is to start the program over. This is a good option for people who have many psychological issues in their lives and need more time to address them and for those who haven't had time to complete the exercises. Restarting also provides clear guidance and structure. It may take a few more weeks of working on the psychological issues and on talking to your mind and your body for the message of MBS to really become integrated and accepted.

If you are a perfectionist, however, it may not be a good idea to restart the program from the beginning. Overly conscientious people with high expectations of themselves may work so hard on the program that it puts added pressure on them, preventing them from getting better. Other people find they are writing about the same psychological issues over and over and feel stuck in a rut. For such people, it is best to take a break from the structured program for a while and follow the rest of the advice in this section.

Another approach is to pick and choose the exercises that you'd like to complete over the next few weeks—those that give you the best opportunity to work on particular issues in ways you find helpful. Feel free to do so, especially if you feel you have made some progress.

What barriers might be preventing you from getting better? Maybe you haven't yet identified some important psychological issues that are causing your mind to continue to produce pain signals. To determine if there are specific barriers you may have missed, review chapters 9 and 10. It's very common for some hidden parts of you to prefer NOT to get better. Identify those potential barriers and complete the writing exercises to address them. You may also need to work on them with the reprogramming the brain affirmations and the meditations.

It's very common for people to have issues in their lives they've avoided addressing, especially ones that make them uncomfortable. Who would want to confront an angry neighbor or boss? Why rehash issues from many years ago with a sister or brother? Wouldn't it be better to forget an issue with a parent or religious leader that goes back all the way to your childhood? What is the benefit of returning to a place where trauma began? And why uncover feelings that are emotionally difficult to deal with?

MBS is often caused by emotions that need to be resolved in order to undo the pain. It's not always enough to write about or meditate on some of these issues. It is frequently necessary to do something actively to resolve them. If this might be the case for you, review chapter 10 and consider beginning this sometimes difficult work. One man had to speak with his father about some issues that had caused tremendous strife many years earlier. Sometimes a difficult decision needs to be made regarding the future of a significant relationship or marriage. A woman found that she had to make a very difficult decision about her son. He had been taking advantage of her for several years, lying and stealing money from her to pay for his drug addiction. She couldn't bring herself to separate from him. But when she did, this is what she wrote:

> "In order to heal yourself from fibromyalgia and other MBS symptoms, you have to look at the truth in your life, no matter what it is. If you live an illusion, you will never reach the end you seek. In this program, I have learned the truth about my life and myself. I have learned things that I needed to learn and have made difficult, yet important, decisions about my life and my relationships. To have health in our bodies, our minds need to be at peace. As I have found peace, I find I like myself more and I find that my body is healthy again. Thanks to this program, my bodily pain, my headaches, and my fatigue are so much better."

On the other hand, if you have already dealt with and processed the stressful and emotional situations in your life, it can be important to stop looking in that direction for your recovery. In that case, going over the same problems or continuing to write about them isn't necessary and can be counter-productive. One of the biggest barriers to getting better is anxiety and fear. You may fear that your symptoms will never get better or that new ones may develop. But if you live in fear, you are more likely to stay in pain and develop new MBS symptoms. Many people have been told by doctors or physical therapists that there is something wrong with their back or neck or joints. They have been warned to be extremely careful in lifting, bending, or running. They live in fear. It is critical to realize that your pain cannot harm you. If you live in fear of pain, you will not get better. You must be able to accept that pain occurs and not panic when it does. You must learn to relax and have confidence that your pain will go away. Know that you are healthy and on the right path. Work to banish worry, fear, and anxiety by using the same techniques that you applied to your pain. Write to the worry, talk to the fear, and meditate on the anxiety.

One woman who had severe pain found that this was a key to getting better. She wrote:

"Something pretty profound happened this last week. The pain nearly went away. I was able to create some wiggle room in my mind to stop thinking about the pain and actually BELIEVE myself capable of being pain-free and VISUALIZE myself engaged in my activity with ease. I did some pretty intense physical exercise with very little symptoms. Some "soreness" was still there the next day, but I nonetheless repeated what I did with courage, not fear, and again, I moved through pretty intense activity with very little discomfort. Why? Trust. All of a sudden, I actually let go. I said to myself, pain or no pain, I am trusting life. If it gives pain, there are still lessons to learn; when I am without pain, it is time to celebrate and be present—not fear what is not there. I also tell myself throughout the day that I am strong, healthy, and at ease in my body—and then visualize my body full of light, moving with grace, confidence and ease. If I shift my attention to my heart and go through my day from a place of trust, no matter how I feel, it is OK. I feel that I can reconnect with trusting life and surrendering. I am practicing those skills (patience, relaxation, gratitude, health) that are the opposite of the traits (worry, fear, distrust) that produce MBS pain."

These are key words to live by: trust, courage, confidence, relaxation, belief, and being comfortable in your own body and in your own life every moment. If you meet fear and anxiety with calmness and ease, and if you know deep down that you are healthy and strong, you will be fine. It takes repetition for the brain to develop new pathways, so you need to keep repeating to yourself: "I am strong and healthy. I can do whatever I choose. I am not afraid. I am confident and calm."

Do as many activities as you can do, and expand them so that you are proving to yourself that you are healthy and strong. One man who had severe pain in both thighs for over twenty years couldn't walk more than ten feet before he had to stop due to excruciating pain. However, he was determined to conquer his pain, and he was absolutely sure that he had MBS and nothing more. He started by walking ten feet and resting—and walking ten more feet. Over the course of a couple of weeks, he could walk fifteen feet, then twenty. As he increased his exercise, his pain became a bit more tolerable, and he realized he was on the right track. He is now pain free and able to walk as much as he likes. Each person needs to figure out how much activity is best and how quickly to increase it. You may want to work with a trainer or take a physical activity class in order to have someone guide you. The more active you are, the quicker you will retrain your brain and develop new non-pain pathways.

For some people, the best thing to do after finishing this program is to take a break from it. The emotional work is significant and can be stressful. Make sure to be kind to yourself and to take time for yourself. It's a critical element in your healing process. If you have not been able to do so, try again to find time for activities for yourself—a minimum of four to five hours per week on fun and pleasurable activities. Keep experimenting until you find something that delights you. It can be walking, riding a bike, knitting, bowling, golf, collecting, shopping, meeting friends for lunch, planning a trip, or anything that gives you joy. If you have to force yourself to do this, it's probably all the more important that you do so.

Another powerful option is to stop focusing on the inward journey and begin to focus more on the external. At some point, it is necessary to balance the hard and long work you've done on your MBS with work for others, for family and community. At times, we can get so wrapped up in our own issues that we neglect to move forward with our lives. So many people have had to put their lives on hold due to chronic pain that a critical element in healing is getting back to living your life. You may decide that you really need to get back to work or exercise or volunteering or connecting to others. These positive, life-affirming activities will help you experience happiness and make contributions to others, as well as yourself. An older woman was living alone and suffering greatly with chronic back pain. After finishing the program, she moved to an assisted living residence and began to engage in new friendships and activities. As she became less isolated and happier, her pain vanished. A middle aged woman with middle and high school children found that while at home, she tended to focus on her symptoms and she just felt worse. She decided to take a part-time job and think less about herself and her symptoms. This was a turning point in her recovery as she felt better when she was engaged in her work.

For some people, it is a matter of persistence. This man continued to work with the program, gradually increasing his trust in himself and his body and gradually increasing his activities.

"It has been about 14-15 months since I started your program and came to see you at your office. At that time, the pain in my hips and back was nonstop and severely limited my activities. I hurt no matter what I was doing. I used to be extremely active, mountain bike racing, skiing, surfing, windsurfing but had given up on ever doing these activities again. I was almost house bound. Since then I have slowly, glacially, improved. I have continued to journal and practice identifying my triggers and to examine issues that are happening in my life. It has been quite a journey of self discovery and I can honestly say that I am a different and better person than I was before the pain started. The progress has been slow, but it does not dominate my life and is inexorably receding. I have continually challenged my pain and have been able to do many things that I truly thought that I'd never do again. Once I convinced myself that the trend would continue to be positive despite the slow pace and frequent backsliding, I became confident enough to overcome the inevitable fear that accompanied these episodes. I have resumed surfing, mountain biking, and taken up kite boarding. I never let the pain stop me from working out, but I went slowly, pushing back the pain envelope. While I am still in some discomfort, my pain continues to recede, but most importantly it doesn't resonate with me emotionally as much anymore. Recently I have been able to envision the light at the end of the tunnel and have been thinking about a "normal life." I recently had enough confidence to finally order a new mountain bike and buy a ski pass."

This program places a great deal of emphasis on reflection and meditation as components of healing. I've been a teacher of mindfulness meditation for more than fifteen years. For people attracted to meditation, I strongly recommend it as a way to continue to investigate and resolve life issues and improve health. Mindfulness meditation can be used throughout the day and is very helpful in dealing with chronic pain (Gardner-Nix, 2009). There are mindfulness meditation teachers all over the world who offer courses and retreats. See www.umassmed.edu/cfm/mbsr to find a program in your area. Ronald Siegel, Psy.D., has an excellent book (*The Mindfulness Solution*, 2010) and a website with several free meditations on it (www.mindfulness-solutions.com).

Another resource I recommend is the work of Byron Katie. She has several books, including *Loving What Is* (2002), and a great website, www.thework.org. Those materials have been invaluable for many of my patients. Several have found relief from their MBS symptoms after viewing her online videos, reading her books, and taking her common-sense advice to heart. Key elements to this work are compassion and forgiveness for oneself and others. Those who have experienced difficult childhoods often feel undeserving of love. They may even blame themselves for being a victim of traumatic events. For people in this situation, recovery from MBS is often dependent on learning love and forgiveness for self. Excellent resources in this regard are *The Mindful Path to Self-Compassion* (Germer, 2009), *The Love Response* (Selhub, 2009), and *Self-Compassion: Stop beating yourself up and leave insecurity behind* (Neff, 2011).

There are also hypnosis and imagery tools that can be extremely helpful. For example, Belleruth Naparstek, Emmett Miller, MD, and several other leaders in the field of mind body medicine have produced CDs that contain visual imagery, relaxation, and hypnotic suggestions designed to calm the mind and allow the body to heal. See www.healthjourneys.com for information on specific CDs that are available for help with healing back pain, headaches, and other forms of Mind Body Syndrome.

Positions of power are expansive, i.e., ones in which you stand, inhale deeply, put your arms up or put your hands on our hips, and move your feet apart to the width of your shoulders. This type of body position leads to changes in your physiology, resulting in increases in testosterone (a power hormone), decreases in cortisol (a stress hormone), and increases in the pain threshold (leading to decreased pain) (Choi, et. al., 2012; Bohns, et. al., 2012). People who assume this type of powerful position for a couple of minutes do better on tests and job interviews than those in submissive positions, such as being curled up in a ball or sitting with head in hands (Carney, et. al., 2010).

There are also a variety of body-based therapies that can help in your recovery, such as yoga, tai chi, Qi gong, and focusing. These activities teach you to move in gentle ways and have more confidence in your body. They teach you to accept sensations in your body in ways that emphasize your power, your ability to move with less pain, your feeling of safety, and feeling comfortable in your own body. As you practice these movements, you will be unlearning the neural pathways of pain, anxiety, and depression. When you combine affirming body movements with affirmations that your body is healthy and strong as you move about in the world, you are reinforcing your wellness and creating a positive cycle of diminished fear, fewer symptoms, and increased confidence in your body and your self.

Finally, many people with persistent MBS symptoms enter into a relationship with a psychologist or counselor that they trust. Individuals with MBS who have depression, anxiety, post-traumatic stress disorder, obsessive-compulsive disorder, eating disorders, and other psychological issues can benefit from counseling and/or medication.

Because the underlying cause of MBS is usually rooted in early childhood emotions, it is very helpful to find a psychologist or therapist who is familiar with these types of problems. Lists of therapists with expertise and interest in MBS can be found at PPDAssociation.org, tmswiki.org, or painreprocessingtherapy.com.Choosing a therapist is an important decision; interview them about their knowledge of MBS prior to engaging in a long-term relationship. Ask if they will read this book or review web sites (see the Appendix) so they know how you'd like to approach your problems.

There are several therapeutic techniques that are designed to help individuals resolve deeper emotional issues. As is obvious from this book, I strongly recommend Intensive Short-Term Dynamic Psychotherapy. Unfortunately, there are relatively few therapists who have been trained in these methods. Dr. Allan Abbass teaches ISTDP or Emotional Awareness and Expression therapies to therapists from his center in Halifax, Nova Scotia. Jon Frederickson, MSW, runs an Institute in Washington, DC and their website has a list of ISTDP practitioners around the world (see www.istd-pInstitute.com). As mentioned earlier, there are many therapists who use similar techniques. Somatic Experiencing is another very useful therapeutic model. This technique was developed by Peter Levine, Ph.D. and there are many practitioners worldwide who work with individuals to unlearn the body's reaction to traumatic experiences (see www.traumahealing.com/somatic-experiencing for more information and a list of practitioners). Another useful "body-centered therapy" is known as Sensori-Motor Integration and was developed by Pat Ogden (sensorimotor-psychotherapy.org). Finally, several patients of mine have found EMDR (Eye Movement Desensitization and Reprocessing; see emdr.com) and EFT (Emotional Freedom Technique; see emofree.com) to be helpful as well. Finally, I can recommend the Internal Family Systems (IFS) approach. This model works very well with the MBS model. In fact, I wrote an article about using IFS for people with mind-body pain, along with Richard Schwartz and Ron Siegel (Siegel, et. al., 2020). You can find more on IFS at ifs-institute.com.

Life coaching is another way that some people learn to resolve their symptoms. There are some coaches who work over the phone or online who are skilled and knowledgeable regarding MBS.

In working with a therapist or coach, continue to explore the relationships between psychological issues and physical events. Our bodies are very sensitive to changes in our minds and reflect those changes on a day-to-day (and even minute-to-minute) basis. When you develop an increase in an MBS symptom or a new MBS symptom, there is a reason for it. Your body speaks to you, but it doesn't have verbal language for communication. It will alert you that something is bothering you by creating a physical (or a psychological) symptom. Listen to it, and discover why it is creating these symptoms whenever they occur. MBS can be viewed as a guide to help you heal your life.

A young woman wrote the following:

"Strange as it may sound, I am thankful for my experience with Mind Body Syndrome. Without the incentive from that wretched pain, I never would have looked inside myself for the answers. In doing so, I was forced to confront old demons and begin the path towards healing, both inside and out."

MBS is treatable and curable. For some, it takes quite awhile and a lot of work. But it is well worth it, so do not give up! The work you do will help you understand yourself and free you from being tied to reactions to emotions. It will help you live the life that you choose to live.

My colleague, Dr. Alicia Batson summarized the key aspects of the treatment of MBS. Look at this list and consider which of these areas might be most important for you to work on.

1. Education about what MBS is and how it works
2. Accepting the diagnosis on both an intellectual level as well as a gut level
3. Learning new ways of interacting with your pain which break the pain-fear-pain cycle
4. Understanding how certain personality traits can, not only be beneficial, but also self-destructive when taken to extremes and turned on the self
5. Learning to recognize, experience and process emotions
6. Learning to think psychologically instead of physically when pain arises (e.g. my arms just started hurting again… what is going on inside emotionally right now?)
7. Learning to stand up for yourself with confidence and self-compassion in the face of life's inevitable stressors
8. Learning to let go of fears and turn towards acceptance and joy in one's life

Once You Have Recovered

Those people who have had dramatic improvements in their MBS symptoms are usually extremely relieved that finally something has worked. They are typically amazed that a relatively simple program could actually take away their pain, and that reactions within the mind could cause their symptoms.

Even if your symptoms are now mild or nonexistent, there are several things you still may want to accomplish. You may want to keep working and learning about yourself. The exercises in this program have proven to be very helpful in dealing with stressful events and emotional reactions. Consider continuing to do them in some way, whether keeping a diary, writing unsent letters or dialogues, or meditating regularly. Use the affirmations and continue to remind yourself that you're healthy, strong, and able to withstand stressful events. Keep this book handy and visible, so that you remember to use these exercises when you need them.

At times, you may develop some amount of recurrent pain or some new MBS symptom. The reason is simple: you are still human. All of our minds and bodies are intimately connected. Since your body serves as a built-in alarm system, it will alert you when things that are occurring in your life are troubling, even if you are not aware that you are upset. Of course, if you get new symptoms, you want to make sure there is nothing physically wrong. You may need to see your doctor to be sure. However, since you understand MBS, you will want to look for issues in your life as a cause for new symptoms. Often it is easy to identify them when you take a few minutes to think. The earlier you identify new symptoms as being due to MBS, the quicker you can stop them from taking hold. Often times, an unsent letter, a meditation, some affirmations, or some exercise can stop new MBS symptoms in their tracks! It is important to remain confident that you are, in fact, healthy and strong and able to conquer any new MBS symptoms. With that attitude, you will be able to maintain freedom from MBS over the long haul.

Finally, you may want to help others. Once you learn about MBS, you will realize that some of your friends and relatives suffer from it. Naturally, you'd like to help them and you'll want to tell them about how their symptoms can be cured if properly understood. However, be forewarned: Most people you tell about this will not be interested, or they will refuse to think that their condition could be MBS. This is a natural consequence of the way that modern medicine approaches physical symptoms. Few doctors are aware of MBS and even fewer patients. Many people's initial reaction to hearing about MBS is that they are being accused of being weak, or crazy, or faking their pain, or that their symptoms are all in their head. They may not understand that people with MBS are just normal people who have emotional reactions to stress.

More doctors and patients need to understand MBS. If they did, many people could be saved from years of suffering, and we would be a healthier society. If there were fewer stigmas attached to the idea that the mind can cause real pain and other symptoms, more people would get the kind of help they really need, rather than receiving medical testing and treatment that is ineffective or even harmful. In addition, health care costs would decline by eliminating unnecessary testing and treatments. You can help by educating your doctor and your friends and family about MBS. In the future, I hope that we will more frequently see this kind of interaction in a doctor's office: "So, I see you've started having back pain (or headaches or stomach pain). I'm going to examine you to make sure there is no sign of a serious medical condition. Then I'd like to ask you a bit about what's been going on in your life."

chapter 12
Frequently Asked Questions

What if pain, the kind that opens a fist, is really the tap of an angel saving us from ourselves? —Mark Nepo

What about asthma, ulcerative colitis, or rheumatoid arthritis? Can these be forms of Mind Body Syndrome?

I generally divide disorders into three categories. Disorders that occur more frequently as people age are primarily degenerative physical conditions, such as cancer, strokes, and heart attacks. Although the mind plays a role in all illnesses, these are not primarily caused by thoughts or emotions, nor can they reliably be cured by changing our thoughts and emotions. A second category of illnesses are those which occur in younger people, have clear evidence of tissue destruction, yet also seem to be significantly influenced by the mind. These disorders include asthma, ulcerative colitis, Crohn's disease, multiple sclerosis, rheumatoid arthritis, and other immune-related disorders. There is no evidence that changing the mind can reliably cure these disorders, and I would not expect that any tissue destruction that has already occurred will be reversed. However, it is possible that this program can help to reduce or eliminate exacerbations of these disorders. It has now been clearly shown that the brain can affect the immune system. In fact, there is a whole field of research known as psycho-neuro-immunology that is devoted to this subject. Therefore, doing the MBS work can not only calm the danger signal, but in some people, also modulate the immune system to turn off auto-immune responses. For people with these auto-immune disorders, it seems reasonable to use a combination of medical treatment and mind-body therapies. The third category of disorder is Mind Body Syndrome in all of its varied manifestations.

I have read that migraine headaches and fibromyalgia are genetic diseases. If that is true, how can they be caused by Mind Body Syndrome?

It is clear that we are not born with a "clean slate." Everyone is born with certain genes for hair, skin, eye color, ability in music and athletics, and general temperament. It has been shown that some people are born with a higher likelihood of being fearful and introverted, while others are more extroverted and risk-taking. Some people have the misfortune to be born with genes that cause them to have specific diseases, such as cystic fibrosis, sickle-cell anemia, or Tay-Sachs disease. Some genes will cause specific disorders, while others simply lead to a higher likelihood of a certain condition. Those genes in the latter group can be "turned on" or "turned off" during our lifetime.

In migraine headaches, fibromyalgia, anxiety, and other disorders that I include under Mind Body Syndrome, genetic factors account for only 15 to 40 percent of the likelihood of developing these disorders. In other words, those genes do not "cause" those disorders, but they can make a person more likely to develop them if they are put in the situation in their life that triggers MBS. The genes associated with MBS will not cause the disorder to occur unless they are turned on by stressful events in childhood and by the occurrence of emotional stressors later in life. The term used for this phenomenon is epigenetics, and a good lay explanation of this can be found in *The Biology of Belief* (Lipton, 2008). When you educate yourself about MBS and take the steps in your life to unlearn your pain, those genes will be turned off.

I get the impression from what I have read that understanding MBS processes is all that is necessary for healing MBS. For me, this does not seem to be enough. Undertanding the process and uncovering the unconscious traumas or stressors seems to be only part of the puzzle, because this has not led to improvement in my symptoms.

In my experience, knowledge about MBS is enough to eliminate pain in approximately 10 to 15 percent of patients. Many other people are able to eliminate MBS symptoms by reducing their level of fear and learning to move forward with their lives. Everyone else needs to figure out how to identify and deal with the psychological issues causing pain. MBS is caused by unresolved emotions, and it is usually necessary to resolve them to get better.

Many people need to make changes in their lives. It often takes a great deal of courage to face the situations that hold us hostage. But we must face those situations and deal with them directly and honestly. While it is true that many situations are unchangeable, we can still cope with them better, understand them better, learn to live with them or accept them, and learn to find the grace and lessons that they teach us. Many situations can be changed, however, and we can make the decisions needed to change them.

Everyone gets pain from time to time. How will I know if a pain is really MBS or something that requires medical attention? Do I need to be concerned that I'll hurt myself if I exercise again?

There is no way to be 100 percent sure if an acute pain is really MBS or an injury. Here are some clues that an acute pain is actually caused by MBS: it occurs without an injury, it occurs when another MBS pain gets better, and/or it occurs after some stress or emotion. For a pain that occurs while running or exercising, it is often hard to know for sure. If it heals within a few days or so, it was probably a mild injury that just needed time to heal. If it persists for a longer time than expected for a mild injury, then it is probably MBS. You can also investigate the symptom to see if it varies with stress, or is inconsistent with a physical injury, like being better or worse at times unrelated to certain movements or activities. If you build up the amount of exercise you do gradually, you should have no problem, as long as you keep reminding your body that it is strong and healthy and that it can tolerate exercise without any problems.

Why is it so important to believe that the program will work? What if I'm skeptical? Will that undermine my likelihood of success?

I'm often a skeptic myself, particularly about expensive medical treatments that don't make biological sense and that make the patient dependent on the doctor. This program is different because it's based on solid scientific research about how pain develops and persists.

All treatment regimens—including exercise, medications, and surgery—work better if the patient believes in them. That's the well-known placebo effect. But this program is more than a placebo. This program works because it addresses the actual underlying reason for the pain. This is just good medicine: finding the source of the problem and dealing with it in a straightforward and powerful manner.

It's fine to have a healthy amount of skepticism. Many people have gotten better despite being skeptical that this program would work for them. But it will be more difficult to be cured if you don't believe that MBS explains why you have your pain. Chronic pain and other MBS symptoms are caused by circuits which have been learned in response to significant emotional issues and have been reinforced over a significant amount of time. These nerve circuits are primarily contained in the subconscious mind and are reinforced by worry, fear, and uncertainty. If you believe a physical problem is causing your pain, this gives the subconscious mind an "out," a way to continue producing pain.

In order to unlearn your pain, you must clearly understand that the source of the pain is due to MBS, that emotional reactions to stress have caused the pain, and that mental processes can reverse the pain. As you engage in this program, you will begin to see how your symptoms vary with changes in your mind, and you will see that your symptoms can improve. As this happens, you will gradually gain the confidence to get better and you will learn to see that MBS is the right diagnosis for your situation.

Should I stop taking my pain medications for this program to work? What about my medication for depression or anxiety?

It is fine to take medication for pain, anxiety, or depression while you are working on the MBS program. If you are in severe pain, it can be very difficult to participate in this program, so pain medications are often necessary. Do not stop any medications without first speaking to your physician. After your pain or anxiety or depression gets better, you can taper off your medication, in consultation with your physician. If you stop your medication too early, your mind can use that as an excuse to cause your MBS symptoms to recur. This is known as the nocebo effect, the opposite of the placebo effect. It is very common for the brain to increase symptoms when fear arises, such as may occur when reducing or stopping a medication. The nocebo effect also occurs when a doctor tells someone that their pain is due to an incurable physical problem, when it's really MBS. Sadly, this occurs all too often. When you do decide to reduce a medication dose, make sure that you remind your brain that lowering the dose will not harm you and that you are safe and confident that you will be OK. This will prevent your brain from activating the nocebo response. If you do notice an increase in symptoms when tapering a medication, you can smile at the brain and calm it using the techniques in this book.

I have been told I need physical therapy in order to stretch and strengthen my body. Should I continue it, or will that deflect attention from the MBS to something "physical?" What about exercise? How much should I do? What about posture?

I encourage all my patients to exercise, get stronger, and learn to trust their bodies. It would be wrong to run on a fractured ankle. But with MBS, there is no fracture and no physical damage, and therefore there should be no fear of injury. What holds people back is pain and fear of pain. So, work through the fear and pain by gradually increasing the amount of exercise that you do.

Physical therapy is a form of exercise, so I have no problem with that. While you are exercising, make sure to tell yourself frequently that your body is strong, you are healthy, there is nothing wrong with your body, and that you are doing this to get stronger. If your physical therapist reinforces the idea that there is something wrong with your muscles or joints, this can delay your recovery from MBS. If you can't find a physical therapist who understands MBS, consider a personal trainer to help you get stronger and more flexible.

Many people are concerned about their posture or the positions that they take while working. A lot of time, effort and money can be spent on getting ergonomically "safe" chairs, desks and other equipment. Studies that have looked at this have found that these concerns are usually way overblown. Our bodies are made to be used and they are not actually damaged by poor posture. It can be uncomfortable to be in one position for an extended period of time, but when you change your posture and move about, the body is reset and any symptoms go away. Persistent symptoms are much more likely to be MBS than due to poor posture.

Some days I have a couple of hours a day to spend on the program, but some days I don't have any time. Is it OK to work on one week's material for two weeks rather than one?

You can go at your own pace. If you can complete the program in two to six months rather than one, that's perfectly fine. I don't want people who are very busy to overwork themselves and put extra stress into their lives. So, find a good balance. But be sure to make time to work on the program so that you get its benefit. You deserve to get better, and you need to take time in order to do the work that's required.

How do I deal with people who doubt the MBS concept? They are always telling me to go to the doctor again to see if there is a physical problem. This makes me doubt myself, and then I find that my pain is worse.

People always do better in the MBS program when they are convinced that their physical and psychological problems are due to stress and reactions to stress. But we will sometimes wonder if we're on the right track. A woman recently told me that she must have something physically wrong because her pain was so severe, even though her pain had lessened after one week of this program. These kinds of doubts are common and will arise in most people.

It is critical to realize that thoughts are uncontrollable. We don't choose what thoughts come into our heads. The mind will continually come up with a wide variety of thoughts, many of which are unproductive, weird, or even inane. If we can't control our own thoughts, we certainly cannot control other people's thoughts, and therefore we must learn ways of reacting to thoughts or else we will be at the mercy of every stray thought that we (or someone else) comes up with. Of course, we also need to deal with emotions, which are often connected to important material from our past.

An excellent way to deal with thoughts and emotions is by practicing mindfulness. The first meditation in chapter 7 provides the basics of mindfulness. This practice teaches us to be aware of thoughts and emotions without having to react to them, without having our bodies react to them, and without allowing the mind to cause pain or other physical symptoms as it has done in the past.

If thoughts (such as doubts) can cause you to have increased pain or other physical symptoms, that confirms that those symptoms are due to MBS. With regard to doubt about having a physical condition, if you have had a good medical evaluation and there are no significant findings on your physical and neurological examination, you most likely have MBS. Your mind is an incredible trickster and will keep you in pain as long as you let it. The solution is to be convinced that you have MBS and to be persistent and believe in yourself, and you'll be fine.

Having discussions with others, such as co-workers, friends and family members, about MBS is often difficult. Most people will simply not understand this approach as it just goes against what most people (and most doctors) believe. So, it's probably a good idea not to discuss this with many people. Of course, you want to get support as you go through the program. If you can identify others who are truly understanding of this approach and caring, you want to meet with them and confide in them. There are online support groups specifically for MBS that can be helpful and meet this need.

I'm just starting my first week of this course and have a question about reprogramming the mind. I think this is a key to my recovery as I've identified some strong triggers that I have not been able to keep from causing my symptoms in the past. Most of the triggers are involved with work, and they make doing my job difficult while also causing me fear. How can I deal with these triggers?

First, it is important to realize that triggers are things that can initiate symptoms, but they are not directly causing them. When Pavlov's dogs salivated at the sound of the buzzer, it triggered the symptoms only because that nerve pathway was learned by their brain. The trigger can be extinguished over time by disconnecting the buzzer from the food. In your case, it would be helpful to figure out why work is a trigger for you. Is it because your symptoms started at work, because you are in, or have been in, difficult situations there, because you do certain activities at work that may seem to cause pain, or all of the above?

Second, you need to look at any issues that are occurring at work and figure out if you can continue to work there and what you can do to change things. If you decide to continue working at this job, you will need to find ways of stopping your pain at work. Persistently talk to yourself prior to going to work, while entering work, and at work. Tell your mind that your body doesn't need to have these symptoms anymore. Get immersed in your job, stay focused on doing the very best you can. Focus on enjoying any aspects of the job that you can, and being grateful for having a job. The more content you are in your situation, the better able you will be to stop the vicious cycle of nerve connections that have formed. If your job is truly not the right place for you at this time, then you can make the decision to find another job and leave. Figure out if that change should happen right away or if you need to delay for a while. Know that you are not trapped and that you have an exit strategy. Remind your brain that you will look out for yourself and take care of yourself. Know that this will not be forever and that you will be able to handle it until you can leave.

Finally, you need to learn to relax and not worry if symptoms develop. The more you worry, the more you will trigger the symptoms, because the symptoms feed on your emotions. You've had symptoms before, and they may be uncomfortable—but they won't harm you, because there is no physical disease. You will survive, and you will get better. Be confident that you are on the mend and getting better. Listen to the first week's meditation and train yourself to accept what is happening now, and learn to let thoughts, emotions, and body sensations go. Then focus on something else, anything else, such as your breath, your elbow, your surroundings, some music, or your work. In this way, you are reprogramming your brain away from the nerve connections that cause symptoms.

After starting the program, I am finding that my symptoms are getting worse. Am I doing something wrong? This has made be anxious, and that seems to make my pain worse. I'm also feeling depressed and tired. Should I stop the program or go slower with it?

It is common for symptoms to become worse or for new symptoms to emerge when starting the program, especially with the writing exercises. There are several reasons for this. First, you are uncovering emotions that have been buried. This is a healthy process, but also one that often leads in the short run to strong feelings, such as worry, fear, sadness, or guilt. Second, your mind is going to realize that you are finally catching onto the fact that the physical symptoms are due to unresolved emotions. Therefore, it will tend to create other symptoms to keep you off track or scare you into stopping this work. The new symptoms can be physical or psychological ones, such as anxiety, fatigue, or depression. You have done nothing wrong; in fact, when this work causes your symptoms to change you are clearly on the right track. Don't give up because this is actually a sign that you are making progress. If you need pain or anxiety medication for the short term, that's fine; don't worry about taking it. You can always stop when you don't need it anymore.

You may also want to consider seeing a counselor. You are absolutely correct that anxiety can cause and exacerbate pain. So, keep writing, meditating, and doing the affirmations. Pain and anxiety are both manifestations of MBS, so treat them the same way. As for depression and fatigue, your mind is trying to give you the message that this work is too hard or too scary. Don't allow your mind to get away with that. Stopping would be giving in to your subconscious mind, which wants to stay in control and avoid change. Write to the negativity and depression; talk to it. Tell it that you know what it's trying to do. As the course progresses, you will begin to overcome those issues, to see them in a new light, to learn from them, and learn to let them go.

I'm either waking up in the middle of the night or I wake up with pain. How can I deal with those things which are occurring while I sleep?

When you sleep, your conscious brain is sleeping, while your subconscious mind is not only awake, but fully in charge. It is necessary to deal with your subconscious in order to stop sleep from being a trigger for your symptoms. Before you go to bed each night, write out a list of the things on your mind and leave it next to the bed (or somewhere else if you prefer). Write at the bottom of the list, "I'll deal with these tomorrow. I will not worry about them at all tonight while I sleep." Then do one of the meditations in this program, a visualization (see chapter 11 for these resources), or listen to some soft music. Finally, before you fall asleep, have a little chat with your brain and its danger signal. Let it know that you're OK and that you're going to be OK; and that there are no major issues that need attending to tonight. Tell your brain that it can keep you awake or wake you up as it pleases, but that you are not afraid of that. You know that you will sleep better over time and that if you don't sleep well tonight, you'll sleep better tomorrow or the next night. Do this each night for two weeks, and you will sleep better and your morning pain will lessen or go away.

As you lie down to go to sleep. Repeat these phrases to yourself: "I know how to fall asleep. I always fall asleep. I will fall asleep. I am fine to stay awake until I do fall asleep." These words will help you to stop trying to fall asleep, since that only makes falling asleep less likely. In fact, the best way to fall asleep is to try to stay awake. So, just relax, stop worrying about sleep and remind yourself that you'll be fine. It may take several nights of not sleeping until your brain calms, but it will as long as you reassure it.

I was doing really well when I started the program. My pain was going down, and I was beginning to feel good for the first time in several years. Then my pain returned, and now it seems worse than ever. What did I do wrong? I'm worried that it won't go away again and that I'll be stuck back where I was. What should I do?

First, you should realize that you have been successful with this program. You saw a decrease in your pain simply by thinking about it differently and beginning to do the psychological exercises. That should reassure you that you can get better.

You should also understand that setbacks do occur in most people. They happen because the brain and the body are deeply interconnected. Subconscious emotions and thoughts can easily trigger pain or other MBS symptoms. You may not even be able to figure out what thoughts or emotions caused the reactivation of pain. You may have started to be more active and then your body said, "Hold on, there; not so fast." The mind and body are used to having pain, and it often takes some time to unlearn the neural circuits that have developed. I still get MBS symptoms at times, and sometimes it is not clear what stress or thoughts bring it on. Here's how to turn it around.

First, be kind to yourself. Don't beat yourself up or blame yourself for this setback. And even though you are in pain, it is critical that you remain certain that MBS is the cause and that you can overcome it. Relax and take some deep breaths; collect yourself; do not let fear overtake you, because that can lead to more pain. Then take some time to try to figure out what triggered the pain. Sometimes, a new stressful situation has arisen or you may think that the work you are doing in this program may lead to changes in relationships that may be difficult to navigate. Sometimes, the danger signal in the brain just falls back into default circuits of pain for a while. Sometimes, the brain ramps up symptoms before they go down, as a temporary reaction to the changes you are making.If you can't, don't worry, just go back to doing the things that led to your initial success. Keep reminding yourself that you are healthy and strong and that this is a temporary setback. Tell yourself that you will be fine soon. Be assertive, and continue to do more physical activities. Do the writing and the meditations. Don't fall into seeing yourself as a victim. Develop confidence in yourself and in your ability to heal yourself. This shall pass, and you will get better.

I am confused about what foods I should eat. I have gotten conflicting information— some say to avoid wheat and dairy products, others say to go organic or vegan. Does food cause or aggravate bodily pains?

Certain people have allergic reactions to specific foods. Testing for wheat allergy (gluten enteropathy) can determine if you should not be eating wheat. Peanut allergic reactions can be life-threatening at times. However, many medical clinicians suggest stopping wheat or dairy or other foods based upon suspect alternative medical testing, such as muscle testing. These tests have not been shown to be accurate. Foods are common "triggers" for MBS and I have seen many people resolve their reactions to foods by simply applying the reprogramming the brain techniques in this book.

Some medical providers suggest that certain foods cause more oxidation in the body leading to free radicals that can cause inflammation. This is true and good health over a lifetime should include healthy eating. However, the type of inflammation that they are talking about is on a very "micro" level. It is my opinion that this level of inflammation does not cause body pain. When inflammation causes body pain, it is a "macro" inflammation, that is, inflammation that is obvious to see upon examination, such as the inflammation that occurs in the joints of people with active rheumatoid arthritis or gout. Macro-inflammation is improved by using anti-inflammatory medications, such as steroids. However, steroids do not help the pain of MBS, which is further evidence that MBS is not due to inflammation. In addition, inflammation is a process that can turn on and off over days, but not seconds or minutes. The pain of MBS can turn on and off within seconds or minutes, which confirms that it is due to neural circuits in the brain and not due to inflammation.

From the MBS point of view, it is important to understand that you can eat whatever you want, whatever feels good, and whatever makes you happy. It will make no difference in pain or MBS. If you are afraid to eat certain foods, that can create MBS symptoms.

This leads me to another point. Many people worry too much. If you worry about what you eat every meal, about what thoughts you have, about whether you wrote or meditated today, you are worrying too much. Everyone has days where they eat better or worse food; days when they think better or "worse" thoughts; engage in writing or meditating more or less. Big deal! Give yourself a break. Realize that no one is perfect and that you can still get better by being imperfect!! In fact, being imperfect is what we are as humans. There are two excellent books on the topic of how understanding our imperfections can lead to less worry and more serenity (Kurtz and Ketcham, 1993; Brown, 2010).

Why does my mind come up with new symptoms when I get rid of one of the old ones? When will it give up?

Once you recognize that the mind often creates substitute symptoms, you will be amazed at the variety of symptoms that may occur. This is a fascinating process to observe. it is very common to see pain move from one area to another or morph into fatigue or OCD symptoms. Most physicians don't understand this process, because it doesn't fit into their purely biomedical view of the body. One woman reported that her physician became angry with her when she reported that her pain kept shifting from one shoulder to the other.

When this process occurs, you can be sure of three things. The diagnosis of MBS is confirmed, because a structural problem in one area would not move around like that. If a particular symptom can disappear for a while that tells you that this symptom can definitely get better. Symptom substitution is a positive sign, as I frequently say: "You've got it on the run!"

The mind will continue to produce new symptoms or substitute symptoms for a variety of reasons. One, it's not quite ready to give up yet. If your symptoms have been there for a long time, it may take a bit longer for the brain to "get the message." Two, you haven't yet integrated the changes that you need to make in your life or in your psyche. Three, you haven't yet accepted yourself fully and completely—you are still fighting yourself, doubting yourself, being afraid of symptoms or of certain issues or events in your life. Four, you haven't yet learned what you need to learn from your symptoms. This may sound odd, but several people in the program have directly asked their symptoms (in meditation or in writing) this question, "What do I need to learn from you?" And finally, the brain can easily fall back into the danger mode just because it is used to doing that. Basically, it is a habit of your brain. Habits can change and your brain will do this less often over time as you continue to calm your brain, remind yourself that you're OK and focus on living the best life that you can.

Don't doubt yourself. You are on the right track. Continue the process of writing, meditating, talking to your brain, and making changes in your life. Almost everyone gets symptom substitution, and if you're able to recognize it quickly and even laugh at the new symptom ("Isn't that funny that my body thinks it can get away with trying that one?"), then you're more likely to rid yourself of MBS symptoms soon.

How do I deal with anxiety? I worry if I'm going to get better and if this pain will come back.

The longer I am involved in this work, the more I see the key relationship between fear, worry, and anxiety and pain. What often happens is that the mind uses anxiety as a symptom substitution—it creates worry and fear when we catch on to the fact that the pain is caused by MBS. This is actually progress, because when anxiety occurs, it means that emotions are less suppressed. Now you can focus on dealing with the fear, worry, and anxiety. Accept that you have these feelings at times; and recognize that there are reasons for them and that they are normal. Then treat the anxiety just as you have learned to treat the pain. Notice it without getting upset, tell it that you know what is causing it, and tell it to go away.

In time, you'll see that the anxiety will begin to lose its power over you; you won't have to fight it or worry that it will cause terrible problems. Listen to the meditation for week one where I talk about noticing thoughts, accepting them as "just thoughts," and letting them go. You can treat fear and anxiety the same way: notice without judging, understand, accept, and let go. The more you feel these feelings without judging them, without fighting them, without worrying that they are a threat, the more you will be able to accept them and let them go. There is also an excellent meditation entitled Stepping into Fear, on Ronald Siegel's website: www.mindfulness-solution.com. Finally, listen to the Embracing Emotions meditation at www.unlearnyourpain.com.

You talk about forgiveness, but isn't that condoning what someone else did?

Forgiveness has little to do with other people. Whether they deserve to be forgiven is irrelevant. If you felt they deserved to be forgiven, you probably would have forgiven them a long time ago. But if you are not able to either forget or forgive, you are allowing the other person to control you and continue to hurt you. So, you are basically deciding to hurt yourself. Is this what you want? Is your anger so important that you will allow it to consume you and continue to cause pain?

Forgiveness doesn't mean that you like what happened, or that you think that was the right thing for someone to do. It means that you accept that it happened. It means that you realize that other people do things for their own reasons and that you have to take care of yourself. It means that you refuse to be controlled or defined by someone else's actions. It means that you are ready to move on and not wallow in anger or defeat. It also means that you realize that the other person was doing the best they could or the only thing they could do at the time.

When you forgive someone, it asserts your power to choose how you think and how you act. It means letting go of the past and learning that you are in control of your thoughts and your life. It is not an act of weakness, but one of strength.

Why do the symptoms of MBS keep coming back after they get better?

Is my mind that persistent?

The answer is "Yes;" your mind is very persistent. In fact, this experience is so common that one should expect that the symptoms will return in one way of another. Here's why.

One way to think of MBS is that it is like a child throwing a temper tantrum. There is a part of our mind that can get very upset and can react violently with little provocation. That child is used to getting his way and keeps it up until the parent capitulates.

The best approach for parents to reduce temper tantrums is to completely ignore the child and not react with fear or worry. However, you wouldn't ignore him unless you know for sure that there is nothing physically wrong; for example, that there is no foreign body in the child's eye. When you know for sure that there is nothing wrong other than the temper tantrum, you can ignore completely and for as long as it takes. This will get the tantrums to stop; but only temporarily at first.

The child will continue to test you. So, every few hours or days, there will be an eruption. Some will be major (this is known as an extinction burst) and some will be minor. This may last for quite a while. It takes time for the new behavior patterns to become engrained.

The same pattern occurs with MBS. You need to know that there is absolutely nothing physically wrong in order to completely ignore the MBS symptoms, which will get them to go away. However, the danger signal in the brain will continue to be activated for a while and from time to time, just like a child's tests. As long as you don't react to new MBS symptoms with fear and worry, you will be able to take control over them and allow them to melt away.

A patient of mine was having some very painful and annoying symptoms in his feet. He recalled a teacher of his who used this phrase when the class was acting up. He would simply say: "I'll wait." My patient said that to his symptoms. He wasn't angry or frustrated; as he knew that the symptoms were simply due to his mind acting up. As he waited without fear, his mind calmed down and the symptoms disappeared.

Finally, as I have stated, you are human and you will always be human. Having some mind-body reactions from time to time is simply part of being human; everyone has them to some degree at some times. I certainly do! If you can accept yourself as being human and not perfect; if you can accept yourself as being OK just as you are; and if you can accept yourself as doing the best that you can, then you will gradually calm the danger signal in your brain and be the person that you were meant to be.

appendix:
additional resources

Books for Understanding and Healing MBS

MEDICAL BOOKS:

The Adaptive Unconscious – Timothy Wilson, PhD

Back in Control: A spine surgeon's roadmap out of chronic pain – David Hanscom, MD

Back Sense – Ronald Siegel, PsyD, Michael Urdang, Douglas Johnson, MD

The Biology of Belief – Bruce Lipton, PhD

Brain Lock – Jeffrey Schwartz, MD

The Brain that Changes Itself – Norman Doidge, MD

Chronic Pain: Your Key to Recovery – Georgie Oldfield, MCSP

Crooked – Cathryn Jakoibson Ramin

The Divided Mind – John Sarno, MD

The Emotional Brain – Joseph LeDoux, PhD

Emotions Revealed – Paul Ekman, PhD

Freedom From Fibromyalgia – Nancy Selfridge, MD

From Paralysis to Fatigue: A History of Psychosomatic Medicine – Edward Shorter, PhD

Hidden From View – Allan Abbass, MD, Howard Schubiner, MD

How Emotions are Made – Lisa Feldman Barrett

The Illusion of Conscious Will – Daniel Wegner, PhD

Internal Family Systems Therapy – Richard Schwartz, PhD and Martha Sweezy, PhD

Lives Transformed: A Revolutionary Method of Dynamic Psychotherapy – David Malan, MD and Patricia Coughlin Della Selva, PhD

The Mindbody Prescription – John Sarno, MD

The Mindful Brain – Daniel Siegel, MD

Overtreated – Shannon Brownlee

Reaching through Resistance – Allan Abbass, MD

Snake Oil Science – R. Barker Bausell, PhD

Stabbed in the Back – Nortin Hadler, MD

Stumbling onto Happiness – Daniel Gilbert, PhD

They Can't Find Anything Wrong – David Clarke, MD

Think Away Your Pain – David Schechter, MD

Train Your Mind, Change Your Brain – Sharon Begley
Unlocking the Unconscious – Habib Davanloo, MD

Watch Your Back: How the Back Pain Industry is Costing Us More and Gving Us Less – Richard A. Deyo, MD

SELF HELP BOOKS:

Don't Panic: Taking Control of Anxiety attacks – Reid Wilson, PhD

Facing the Fire – John Lee

The Feeling Good Handbook – David Burns, MD.

Forgive for Good: A Proven Prescription for Health and Happiness – Fred Luskin, PhD

Full Catastrophe Living – Jon Kabat-Zinn, PhD

The Gifts of Imperfection: Let Go of Who You Think You're Supposed to Be and Embrace Who You Are – Brené Brown, PhD

The Journey: A Practical Guide to Healing Your Life and Setting Yourself Free – Brandon Bays

The Love Response – Eva Selhub, MD

Loving What Is – Byron Katie

Man's Search for Meaning – Viktor Frankl, MD

The Mindfulness Path to Self-Compassion – Christopher Germer, PhD

The Mindfulness Solution – Ronald Siegel, PsyD

The Places that Scare You – Pema Chodron

The Power of Now – Eckhart Tolle

The Presence Process – Michael Brown

Sanity, Insanity, and Common Sense – Enrique Suarez

The Secret Code of Success – Noah St. John

Self-Compassion: Stop Beating Yourself Up and Leave Insecurity Behind – Kristin Neff, PhD

Slowing Down to the Speed of Life – Joe Bailey

The Spirituality of Imperfection: Storytelling and the Search for Meaning – Ernest Kurtz and Katherine Ketcham

Waking the Tiger: Healing Trauma – Peter Levine

What to Say When You Talk to Yourself – Shad Helmstetter

You Can Be Happy No Matter What – Richard Carlson

Websites and Blogs:

Allan Abbass, MD: istdp.ca

David Clarke, MD: stressillness.com

Emotional Freedom Technique: emofree.com

Eye Movement Desensitization and Reprocessing: emdr.com

Health Journeys: healthjourneys.com

IFS Institute: selfleadership.com

ISTDP Institute: istdpInstitute.com

Byron Katie: thework.org

Pat Ogden, PhD: sensorimotorpsychotherapy.org

Peter Levine, PhD: traumahealing.com/somatic-experiencing

PRT Institute: painreprocessing-therapy.com

PPD/TMS Peer Network: tmswiki.org

Psychophysiologic Disorders Association: ppdassociation.org

John Sarno, MD: www.thankyoudrsarno.com

Howard Schubiner, MD: unlearnyourpain.com

Ronald Siegel, PsyD: mindfulness-solution.com

Marc Sopher, MD: tms-mindbodymedicine.com

David Schechter, MD: mindbodymedicine.com

TMS Help Forum: tmshelp.com

University of Massachusetts Center on Mindfulness: www.umassmed.edu/cfm/mbsr

references

Aaron RV, Finan PH, Wegener ST, Keefe FJ, and Lumley MA. Emotion regulation as a transdiagnostic factor underlying co-occurring chronic pain and problematic opioid use. *American Psychologist*, 2020, 75: 796-810.

Abbass A. Intensive short-term dynamic psychotherapy in a private psychiatric office: Clinical and cost effectiveness. *American Journal of Psychotherapy*. 2002, 56: 225-232.

Abbass A. Short-term dynamic therapies in the treatment of major of depression. *Canadian Journal of Psychotherapy*. 2002, 47: 193.

Abbass A. The cost-effectiveness of short-term dynamic psychotherapy. *Journal of Pharmacoeconomics and Outcomes Research*. 2003, 3: 535-539.

Abbass A, Lovas D, Purdy A. Direct diagnosis and management of emotional factors in the chronic headache patient. *Cephalalgia*. 2008, 28: 1305–1314.

Abbass A, Kisely S, Kroenke K. Short-term Psychodynamic Psychotherapy for Somatic Symptom Disorders: A systematic review and meta-analysis. *Psychotherapy and Psychosomatics*. 2009, 78: 265–274.

Abbass A, Campbell S, Magee K, Tarzwell R. Intensive short-term dynamic psychotherapy to reduce rates of emergency department return visits for patients with medically unexplained symptoms: preliminary evidence from a pre-post intervention study. *Canadian Journal of Emergency Medicine*. 2009, 11: 529-34.

Abbass A, Campbell S, Magee K, Lenzer I and Hann G, Tarzwell R. Cost Savings of Treatment of Medically Unexplained Symptoms Using Intensive Short-term Dynamic Psychotherapy (ISTDP) by a Hospital Emergency Department. *Archives of Medical Psychology*. 2010, 2: 34-44.

Abbass A, Campbell S, Hann G, Lenzer I, Tarzwell R. Implementing an Emotion-Focused Consultation Service to Examine Medically Unexplained Symptoms in the Emergency Department. *Archives of Medical Psychology*. 2010, 2: 44-52.

Abbass A. *Reaching through Resistance: Advanced Psychotherapy Techniques*. Seven Leaves Press, Kansas City, MO. 2015.

Amir M, Kaplan Z, Neumann L, Sharabani R, Shani N, Buskila D. Post-traumatic stress disorder, tenderness and fibromyalgia. *Journal of Psychosomatic Research*. 1997, 42: 607-613.

Anda RF, Felitti VJ, Bremner JD, Walker JD, Whitfield C, Perry BD, Dube SR, Giles WH. The enduring effects of abuse and related adverse experiences in childhood: A convergence of evidence from neurobiology and epidemiology. *European Archives of Psychiatry and Clinical Neuroscience*. 2006, 256: 174-86.

Arborelius L, Eklund MB. Both long and brief maternal separation produces persistent changes in tissue levels of brain monoamines in middle-aged female rats. *Neuroscience*. 2007, 145: 738-750.

Arkowitz H, Lilienfeld SO. Why science tells us not to rely on eye witness accounts. *Scientific American Mind*. January 1, 2010.

Ashar YK, Gordon A, Schubiner H, Uipi C, et. al., Lumley MA, Wager TD. Pain Reprocessing Therapy for Chronic Back Pain: A Randomized Controlled Trial with Functional Neuroimaging. *JAMA Psychiatry*. 2022;79(1):13–23.

Asmundson GJG, Katz J. Understanding the co-occurrence of anxiety disorders and chronic pain: State of the art. *Depression and Anxiety*. 2009, 26: 888-901.

Assor A, Roth G, Deci EL. The emotional costs of parents' conditional regard: A self-determination theory analysis. *Journal of Personality*. 2004, 72: 47-88.

Bailey KM, Carleton RN, Ylaeyen JWS, Asmundson GJG. Treatments addressing pain-related fear and anxiety in patients with chronic musculoskeletal pain: A preliminary review. *Cognitive Behaviour Therapy*. 2009, epub. August 20, 2009.

Baliki, MN, Geha PY, Apkarian AV, Chialvo DR. Beyond Feeling: Chronic Pain Hurts the Brain, Disrupting the Default-Mode Network Dynamics. *The Journal of Neuro- science.* 2008, 28: 1398-1403.

Bandura A. *Self-efficacy: The Exercise of Control.* W. H. Freeman, New York, NY. 1997.

Bargh JA, Pietromonaco P. Automatic information processing and social perception: The influence of trait information presented outside of conscious awareness on impression formation. *Journal of Personality and Social Psychology.* 1982, 43: 437-449.

Bargh JA. Auto-motives: Preconscious determinants of social interaction. In *Handbook of Motivation and Cognition,* T. Higgins and R. M. Sorrentino (eds.). Guilford Press. New York, NY. 1990.

Bargh JA, Chen M, Burrows L. Automaticity of social behavior: Direct effects of trait construct and stereotype activation on action. *Journal of Personality and Social Psychology.* 1996, 71: 230-244.

Barrett, L. *How emotions are made: The secret life of the brain.* Houghton Mifflin Harcourt, Boston, New York, 2017.

Barrett L and Simmons WK. Interoceptive predictions in the brain. *Nature Reviews Neuroscience.* 2015, 16: 419-429.

Baumgartner E, Finckh A, Cedraschi C, Vischer T. A six year prospective study of a cohort of patients with fibromyalgia. *Annals of Rheumatologic Diseases.* 2002, 61: 644-5.

Bausell, RB. *Snake Oil Science: The truth about complementary and alternative medicine.* Oxford University Press, New York, NY. 2007.

Beckham JC, Crawford AL, Feldman ME, Kirby AC, Hertzberg MA, Davidson JR, Moore SD. Chronic posttraumatic stress disorder and chronic pain in Vietnam combat veterans. *Journal of Psychosomatic Research.* 1997, 43: 379-389.

Begley S. *Train Your Mind, Change Your Brain.* Random House, New York, NY. 2008.

Bohns VK, Wiltermuth SS. It hurts when I do this (or you do that): Posture and pain tolerance. *Journal of Experimental Social Psychology.* 2012, 48: 341-345.

Boos N, Semmer N, Elfering A, Schade V, Gal I, Zanetti M, Kissling R, Buchegger N, Hodler J, Main CJ. Natural history of individuals with asymptomatic disc abnormalities in magnetic resonance imaging: predictors of low back pain-related medical consultation and work incapacity. *Spine.* 2000, 25: 1484-92.

Bornstein, RF. Reconnecting psychoanalysis to mainstream psychology. Challenges and opportunities. *Psychoanalytic Psychology.* 2005, 22: 323–340.

Borenstein DG, O'Mara JW Jr, Boden SD, Lauerman WC, Jacobson A, Platenberg C, Schellinger D, Wiesel SW. The value of magnetic resonance imaging of the lumbar spine to predict low-back pain in asymptomatic subjects: a seven-year follow-up study. *Journal of Bone and Joint Surgery (American)* 2001, 83-A: 1306-11.

Brinjikji W, Luetmer PH, Comstock B, Bresnahan BW, Chen LE, Deyo RA, Halabi S, Turner JA, Avins AL, James K, Wald JT, Kallmes DF, Jarvik JG. Systematic literature review of imaging features of spinal degeneration in asymptomatic populations. *American Journal of Neuroradiology.* 2015, 36: 811-6.

Brody H and Brody D. *The Placebo Response: How you can release the body's inner pharmacy.* HarperCollins Publishers, New York, NY. 2001.

Brown, B. *The gifts of imperfection: Let go of who you think you're supposed to be and embrace who you are.* Hazelden Press, Center City, MN. 2010.

Brown S, Vaughan C. *Play: How it Shapes the Brain, Opens the Imagination, and Invigorates the Soul.* Penguin Books, New York. 2009.

Brownlee S. *Overtreated: Why too much medicine is making us sicker and poorer.* Bloomsbury USA, New York, NY. 2007.

Burger AJ, Lumley MA, Carty JN, Latsch DV, Thakur ER, Hyde-Nolan ME, Hijazi AM, Schubiner H. The effects of a novel psychological attribution and emotional awareness and expression therapy for chronic musculoskeletal pain: A preliminary, uncontrolled trial. *Journal of Psychosomatic Research.* 2016, 81: 1-8.

Burns D. *The Feeling Good Handbook.* Penguin Putnam, New York, NY. 1999.
Burns JW. Arousal of negative emotions and symptom-specific reactivity in chronic low back pain patients. *Emotion.* 2006, 6: 309-19.

Burns JW, Quartana P, Gilliam W, Gray E, Matsuura J, Nappi C, Wolfe B, Lofland K. Effects of anger suppression on pain severity and pain behaviors among chronic pain patients: evaluation of an ironic process model. *Health Psychology.* 2008, 27: 645-652.

Butler D, Moseley L. *Explain Pain. Orthopedic Physical Therapy Products.* Minneapolis, MN. 2003.

Carney DR, Cuddy AJC, Yap AJ. Power posing: Brief nonverbal displays affect neuroendocrine levels and risk tolerance. *Psychological Science.* 2010, 21: 1363-1368.

Carragee EJ. Clinical practice. Persistent low back pain. *New England Journal of Medicine.* 2005, 352: 1891-8.

Cascio CN, O'Donnell MB, Tinney FJ, et. al. Self-affirmation activates brain systems associated with self-related processing and reward and is reinforced by future orientation. *Social Cognitive and Affective Neuroscience*, 2016, 11: 621–629.

Castro WH, Meyer SJ, Becke ME, Nentwig CG, Hein MF, Ercan BI, Thomann S, Wessels U, Du Chesne AE. No stress—no whiplash? Prevalence of "whiplash" symptoms following exposure to a placebo rear-end collision. *Interna- tional Journal of Legal Medicine.* 2001, 114: 316-22.

Celiker R, Borman P, Oktem F, Gokce-Kutsal Y, Basgoze O. Psychological disturbance in fibromyalgia: relation to pain severity. *Clinical Rheumatology.* 1997, 16: 179-184.

Choi JC, Chung MI, Lee YD. Modulation of pain sensation by stress-related testosterone and cortisol. *Anesthesia.* 2012, 67: 1146-1151.

Chou R, Stanos SP, Rosenquist RW. Nonsurgical interven- tional therapies for low back pain: a review of the evidence for an American Pain Society clinical practice guideline. *Spine* (Phila PA, 1976). 2009, 34: 1078-1093.

Christakis NA and Fowler JH. The spread of obesity in a large social network over 32 years. *New England Journal of Medicine.* 2007, 357: 370-379.

Christakis NA and Fowler JH. The collective dynamics of smoking in a large social network. *New England Journal of Medicine.* 2008, 358: 2249-2258.

Clarke DD. T*hey can't find anything wrong: 7 keys to understanding, treating, and healing stress.* First Sentient Publications, Boulder, CO. 2007.

Cohen N, Ader R, Green N, Bovbjerg D. Conditioned suppression of a thymus-independent antibody response. *Psychosomatic Medicine.* 1979, 41: 487-91.

Cohen H, Neumann L, Haiman Y, Matar MA, Buskila D. Prevalence of post-traumatic stress disorder in fibromyal- gia patients: overlapping syndrome or post-traumatic fibromyalgia syndrome? *Seminars in Arthritis and Rheumatism.* 2002, 32: 38-50.

Costa PT Jr, Terracciano A, McCrae RR. Gender differences in personality traits across cultures: robust and surprising findings. *Journal of Personality and Social Psychology.* 2001, 81: 322-31.

Crombag HFM, Wagenaar WA, van Koppen PJ. Crashing memories and the problem of 'source monitoring.' *Applied Cognitive Psychology.* 1996,10: 95–104.

Crum A, Salovey P, and Achor S. Rethinking Stress: The Role of Mindsets in Determining the Stress Response. *Journal of Personality and Social Psychology.* 2013, 104: 716-733.

Crum AJ, Langer EJ. Mind-set matters: exercise and the placebo effect. *Psychological Science.* 2007, 18: 165-171.

Cunningham A. Ivan Pavlov and the conditioning of physiological responses. *Advances in Mind Body Medicine.* 2001, 17: 7-8.

Das P, Kemp AH, Liddell BJ, Brown KJ, Olivier G, Peduto A, Gordon E, Williams LM. Pathways for fear perception: modulation of amygdala activity by thalamo-cortical systems. *Neuroimage.* 2005, 26: 141-148.

Davanloo H. *Basic Principles and Techniques in Short-Term Dynamic Psychotherapy.* Spectrum Press, New York, NY. 1978.

Davanloo H. *Unlocking the Unconscious.* Wiley Press, New York, NY. 1990.

Davanloo H. Intensive short-term dynamic psychother- apy—central dynamic sequences. *International Journal of Intensive Short-Term Dynamic Psychotherapy.* 1999, 13: 211-236 and 237–262.

Derbyshire SWG, Whalley MG, Stenger VA, Oakley DA. Cerebral activation during hypnotically induced and imagined pain. *Neuroimage.* 2004, 23: 392– 401.

Deyo RA, Rainville J, Kent DL. What can the history and physical examination tell us about low back pain? *Journal of the American Medical Association.* 1992, 268: 760-5.

Deyo RA, Mirza SK, Turner JA, Martin BI. Overtreating chronic back pain: time to back off? *Journal of the American Board of Family Medicine.* 2009, 22: 62-8.

Deyo RA. *Watch Your Back: How the back pain industry is costing us more and giving us less.* Cornell University Press, Ithaca, NY. 2015.

Doidge N. *The Brain that Changes Itself.* Penguin Books, New York, NY. 2007.

Donnino MW, Thompson GS, Mehtab S, et. al. Psychophysiologic symptom relief therapy for chronic back pain: a pilot randomized controlled trial. *Pain Reports,* 2021, 6: e959.

Drew T, Vo MLH, Wolfe, JM. The invisible gorilla strikes again: Sustained inattentional blindness in expert observers. *Psychological Science.* 2013, 24: 1848-1853.

Duhigg C. *The Power of Habit: Why we do what we do in life and business.* Random House, New York, NY. 2012.

Eisenberger NI, Jarcho JM,Lieberman MD, Naliboff BD. An experimental study of shared sensitivity to physical pain and social rejection. *Pain.* 2006, 126: 132-138.

Eisenberger NI, Lieberman MD, Williams KD. Does rejection hurt? An fMRI study of social exclusion. *Science.* 2003, 302: 290-292.

Enright RD. *Forgiveness is a choice.* American Psychologi- cal Association, Washington, DC. 2001.

Ferrari R, Russell AS. Effect of a symptom diary on symptom frequency and intensity in healthy subjects. *Journal of Rheumatology.* 2010, 37: 2386-2387.

Ferrari R. Effect of a pain diary use on recovery from acute low back pain (lumbar) sprain. *Rheumatology International.* 2015, 35: 55-59.

Ferrari R, Louw D. Effect of a pain diary use on recovery from acute whiplash injury: a cohort study. *Journal of Zhejiang University, Science B.* 2013, 14: 1049-1053.

Fisher JP, Hassan DT, O'Connor. Minerva. *British Medical Journal.* 1995, 310: 70.

Fitzgerald KD, Welsh RC, Gehring WJ, Abelson JL, Himle JA, Liberzon I, Taylor SF. Error-related hyperactivity of the anterior cingulate cortex in obsessive-compulsive disorder. *Biological Psychiatry.* 2005, 57: 287-94.

Flor H, Elbert T, Knecht S, Wienbruch C, Pantev C, Birbaumer N, Larbig W, Taub E. Phantom-limb pain as a perceptual correlate of cortical reorganization following arm amputation. *Nature.* 1995, 375: 482-4.

Fowler JH and Christakis NA. The dynamic spread of happiness in a large social network: longitudinal analysis over 20 years in the Framingham heart study. *British Medical Journal.* 2008, 337: a2338.

Frankl V. *Man's Search for Meaning.* Beacon Press, Boston, MA. 2000 (originally published in 1946).

Freud S, Strachey J. *Sigmund Freud: The ego and the id.* W. W. Norton and Co., New York, NY. 1960.

Friedly JL, Comstock BA, Turner JA, et. al. A randomized trial of epidural glucocorticoid injections for spinal stenosis. *New England Journal of Medicine.* 2014, 371: 11-21.

Gardner-Nix J. *The Mindfulness Solution to Pain: Step-by-step techniques for chronic pain management.* New Harbinger Publications, Oakland, CA. 2009.

Gatchel RJ, Polatin PB, Mayer TG. The dominant role of psychosocial risk factors in the development of chronic low back pain disability. *Spine.* 1995, 20: 2702-9.

Geisser ME, Strader Donnell C, Petzke F, Gracely RH, Clauw DJ, Williams DA. Comorbid somatic symptoms and functional status in patients with fibromyalgia and chronic fatigue syndrome: sensory amplification as a common mechanism. *Psychosomatics.* 2008, 49: 235-42.

Germer C. *The Mindful Path to Self-Compassion: Freeing yourself from destructive thoughts and emotions.* The Guilford Press, New York, NY. 2009.

Goebel MU, Trebst AE, Steiner J, Xie YF, Exton MS, Frede S, Canbay AE, Michel MC, Heemann U, Schedlowski M. Behavioral conditioning of immunosuppression is possible in humans. *Federation of American Societies for Experimental Biology Journal.* 2002, 16: 1869-73.

Goldberg N. *Writing Down the Bones: Freeing the writer within.* Shambala Press, Boston, MA. 1986.

Goldberg RT, Pachas WN, Keith D. Relationship between traumatic events in childhood and chronic pain. *Disability and Rehabilitation.* 1999, 21: 23-30.

Goldenberg DL, Burckhardt C, Crofford L. Management of fibromyalgia syndrome. *Journal of the American Medical Association.* 2004, 292: 2388-95.

Gordon A, Ziv A. *The Way Out: A revolutionary, scientifically proven approach to healing chronic pain.* Avery Books, Penguin Random House, New York, 2021.

Gracely RH, Petzke F, Wolf JM, Clauw DJ. Functional magnetic resonance imaging evidence of augmented pain processing in fibromyalgia. *Arthritis and Rheumatism.* 2002, 46: 1333-43.

Grossman P, Tiefenthaler-Gilmer U, Raysz A, Kesper U. Mindfulness training as an intervention for fibromyalgia: evidence of postintervention and 3-year follow-up benefits in well-being. *Psychotherapy and Psychosomatics.* 2007, 76: 226-233.

Hanscom D. *Back in Control: A spine surgeon's roadmap out of chronic pain.* Vertus Press, Seattle, WA. 2012.

Harriman PL. A case of hysterical paralysis. *Journal of Abnormal Psychology.* 1935, 29: 455-456.

Hebb DO. *The organization of behavior.* New York: Wiley & Sons, 1949.

Hensche N, Maher CG, Refshauge KM, Herbert RD, Cumming RG, Bleasel J, York J, Das A, McAuley JH. Prevalence of and screening for serious spinal pathology in patients presenting to primary care settings with acute low back pain. *Arthritis and Rheumatism.* 2009, 60: 3072-3080.

Hill PL, Turiano NA. Purpose in life as a predictor of mortality across adulthood. *Psychological Science.* 2014, 25: 1482-1486.

Holt-Lunstad J, Smith TB, Layton JB. Social relationships and mortality risk: a meta-analytic review. *Public Library of Science Medicine.* 2010, 7:e1000316. doi: 10.1371/journal.pmed.1000316.

Hooley JM, Gruber SA, Scott LA, Hiller JB, Yurgelun-Todd DA. Activation in dorsolateral prefrontal cortex in response to maternal criticism and praise in recovered depressed and healthy control participants. *Biological Psychiatry.* 2005, 57: 809-12.

Hsu MC, Schubiner H, Lumley MA, Stracks JS, Clauw DJ, Williams DA. Sustained pain reduction through affective self-awareness in fibromyalgia: a randomized controlled trial. *Journal of General Internal Medicine.* 2010, 25: 1064-70.

Illich I. *Medical nemesis: the expropriation of health.* Pantheon Press, New York, NY. 1976.

Institute of Medicine. *Relieving Pain in America: A Blueprint for Transforming Prevention, Care, Education, and Research.* Consensus Report, National Academy of Sciences. July 29, 2011.

James, W. What is an emotion? *Mind.* 1884, 9: 188-205.

Jensen MC, Brant-Zawadzki MN, Obuchowski N, Modic MT, Malkasian D, Ross JS. Magnetic resonance imaging of the lumbar spine in people without back pain. *New England Journal of Medicine.* 1994, 331: 69-73.

Kabat-Zinn J. An outpatient program in behavioral medi- cine for chronic pain patients based on the practice of mindfulness meditation: Theoretical considerations and preliminary results. *General Hospital Psychiatry.* 1982, 4: 33-47.

Katie B. *Loving What Is.* Three Rivers Press, New York, NY. 2002.

Keller RB, Atlas SJ, Soule DN, Singer DE, Deyo RA. Relationship between rates and outcomes of operative treatment for lumbar disc herniation and spinal stenosis. *Journal of Bone and Joint Surgery.* 1999, 81: 752-762.

Kirsch, I. Response expectancy as a determinant of experience and behavior. *American Psychologist.* 1985, 11: 1189-1202.

Kivimaki M, Leino-Arjas P, Virtanen M, Elovainio M, Keltikangas-Jarvinen L, Puttonen S, Vartia M, Brunner E, Vahtera J. Work stress and incidence of newly diagnosed fibromyalgia. *Journal of Psychosomatic Research.* 2004, 57: 417-422.

Knight DC, Nguyen HT, Bandetti PA. Expression of conditional fear with and without awareness. *Proceedings of the National Academy of Sciences of the USA.* 2003, 25: 15280-15283.

Kross E, Berman, MG, Mischel W, Smith EE, Wager, TD. Social rejection shares somatosensory representations with physical pain. *Proceedings of the National Academy of Sciences of the USA.* 2011, 108: 6270-6275.

Kurtz E, Ketcham K. *The spirituality of imperfection.* Bantam Books, New York, NY. 1992.

Lacourse MG, Orr EL, Cramer SC, Cohen MJ. Brain activation during execution and motor imagery of novel and skilled sequential hand movements. *Neuroimage.* 2005, 27: 505-19.

Lange G, DeLuca J, Maldjian JA, Lee HJ, Tiersky LA, Natelson BH. Brain MRI abnormalities exist in a subset of patients with chronic fatigue syndrome. *Journal of the Neurological Sciences.* 1999, 171: 3-7.

LeDoux J. *The Emotional Brain: The mysterious underpinnings of emotional life.* Touchstone Books, Simon and Schuster, New York, NY. 1996.

Levenson RW. Autonomic nervous system differences among emotions. *Psychological Science.* 1992, 3: 23-31.

Lieberman MD, Jarcho JM, Berman S, Naliboff BD, Suyenobu BY, Mandelkern M, Mayer EA. The neural correlates of placebo effects: a disruption account. *NeuroImage.* 2004, 22: 447–455.

Lipton BH. *The Biology of Belief.* Hay House Inc., Carlsbad, CA. 2008.

Lum TE, Fairbanks RJ, Pennington EC, Zwemet FL. Profiles in patient safety: Misplaced femoral line guidewire and multiple failures to detect the foreign body on chest radiography. *Academic Emergency Medicine.* 2005, 12: 658-662.

Lumley MA, Cohen JL, Borszcz GS, Cano A, Radcliffe AM, Porter LS, Schubiner H, Keefe FJ. Pain and emotion: a biopsychosocial review of recent research. *Journal of Clinical Psychology.* 2011, 67: 942-68.

Lumley MA, Schubiner H, Lockhart NA, et. al. Emotional awareness and expression therapy, cognitive-behavioral therapy, and education for fibromyalgia: A cluster-randomized, controlled trial. *PAIN.* 2017, 158: 2354-2363.

Luskin F. *Forgive for Good: A proven prescription for health and happiness.* HarperCollins Publishers, New York, NY. 2002.

MacIver K, Lloyd DM, Kelly S, Roberts N, Nurmikko T. Phantom limb pain, cortical reorganization and the therapeutic effect of mental imagery. *Brain.* 2008, 131: 2181-91.

Malan D and Selva PCD. *Lives Transformed: A revolutionary method of dynamic psychotherapy.* Karnac Books, London, UK. 2006.

Malik H, Lovell M. Soft tissue neck symptoms following high-energy road traffic accidents. *Spine.* 2004, 29: E315-7.

Martin BI, Deyo RA, Mirza SK, Turner JA, Comstock BA, Hollingworth W, Sullivan SD. Expenditures and health status among adults with back and neck problems. *Journal of the American Medical Association.* 2008, 299: 656-664.

Matta J, Wiernik E, Robineau O, et al. Association of Self-reported COVID-19 Infection and SARS-CoV-2 Serology Test Results With Persistent Physical Symptoms Among French Adults During the COVID-19 Pandemic. *JAMA Intern Med.* 2022;182(1):19–25. doi:10.1001/jamainternmed.2021.6454

May A. Chronic pain may change the structure of the brain. *Pain.* 2008, 137: 7-15.

McBeth J, Silman AJ, Gupta A, Chiu YH, Ray D, Morriss R, Dickens C, King Y, Macfarlane GJ. Moderation of psychosocial risk factors through dysfunction of the hypothalamic-pituitary-adrenal stress axis in the onset of chronic widespread musculoskeletal pain: findings of a population-based prospective cohort study. *Arthritis and Rheumatism.* 2007, 56: 360-71.

McCullough ME, Pargament KI, Thoresen CE (eds.). *Forgiveness: Theory, Research and Practice.* Guilford Press, New York, NY. 2001.

McEwen BS. Stress, adaptation, and disease: Allostasis and allostatic load. *Annals of the New York Academy of Sciences.* 1998, 840: 33-44.

Melzack R, Casey KL. Sensory, motivational and central control determinants of pain. InKenshalo DR (ed.), *The Skin Senses.* Charles C. Thomas Publishing, Springfield, IL. 1968.

Mitra S. Opioid-induced hyperalgesia: pathophysiology and clinical implications. *Journal of Opioid Management.* 2008, 4: 123-130.

Moseley GL, Zalucki N, Birklein F, Marinus J, van Hilten JJ, Luomajoki H. Thinking about movement hurts: the effect of motor imagery on pain and swelling in people with chronic arm pain. *Arthritis and Rheumatism.* 2008, 59: 623-31.

Moseley L. *Painful Yarns.* Orthopedic Physical Therapy Products. Minneapolis, MN. 2007.

Murray CJL and the US Burden of Disease Collaboration. The State of US Health, 1990-2010: Burden of Diseases, Injuries, and Risk Factors. *JAMA.* 2013, 310: 591-608.

Neff K. *Self-Compassion: Stop beating yourself up and leave insecurity behind.* HarperCollins Publishers, New York, NY. 2011.

Nabi H, Kivimäki M, Batty GD, Shipley MJ, et. al. Increased risk of coronary heart disease among individuals reporting adverse impact of stress on their health: the Whitehall II prospective cohort study. *European Heart Journal.* 2013. doi:10.1093/eurheartj/eht216.

Nguyen TH, Randolph DC, Talmage J, Succop P, Travis R. Long-term outcomes of lumbar fusion among workers' compensation subjects: a historical cohort study. *Spine.* 2011, 36: 320-31.

Noakes, TD. *Lore of Running.* Oxford University Press Southern Africa. 2003.

Nunn KP, Lask B, Owen I. Pervasive refusal syndrome (PRS) 21 years on: a re-conceptualisation and a renaming. *European Child and Adolescent Psychiatry.* 2014, 23: 163–172.

Ochsner KN, Zaki J, Hamelin J, Ludlow DH, Knierim K, Ramachandran T, Glover GH, Mackey SC. Your pain or mine? Common and distinct neural systems supporting the perception of pain in self and other. *Social Cognitive and Affective Neuroscience.* 2008, 3:144-160.

Ohman A. Fear and anxiety as emotional phenomena: Clinical, phenomenological, evolutionary perspectives, and information-processing mechanisms. *In Handbook of the emotions*, M. Lewis and J.M. Haviland (eds.), Guilford Press, New York, NY. 1992.

Okifuji A, Turk DC. Stress and psychophysiological dysregulation in patients with fibromyalgia syndrome. *Applied Psychophysiology and Biofeedback.* 2002, 27: 129-140.

O'Sullivan S. *The sleeping beauties: And other stories of mystery illness.* Pantheon Books, New York, 2021.

Paquette V, Lévesque J, Mensour B, Leroux JM, Beaudoin G, Bourgouin P, Beauregard M. Change the mind and you change the brain: Effects of cognitive-behavioral therapy on the neural correlates of spider phobia. *NeuroImage.* 2003, 18: 401-409.

Paul E, Fancourt D. Does pre-infection stress increase he risk of long COVID? Longitudinal associations between adversity worries and experiences in the month prior to COVID-19 infection and the development of long COVID and specific long COVID symptoms. In press, 2022.

Pennebaker J. *Writing to Heal: A guided journey to recovering from trauma and emotional upheaval.* New Harbinger Publications, Inc. Oakland, CA. 2004.

Pennebaker J. *Opening Up: The healing power of expressing emotions.* Guilford Press, New York, NY. 1990.

Ploner M, Freund HJ, Schnitzler A. Pain affect without pain sensation in a patient with a postcentral lesion. *Pain.* 1999, 81: 211-214.

Progoff I. *At a Journal Workshop: The Basic Text and Guide for Using the Intensive Journal Process.* Dialogue House Library, New York, NY. 1975.

Quartana PJ, Burns JW. Painful consequences of anger suppression. *Emotion.* 2007, 7: 400-14.

Quoidbach J, Gruber J, Mikolajczak M, Kogan A, Kotsou I, Norton MI. Emodiversity and emotional ecosystem. *Journal of Experimental Psychology: General.* 2014, 143: 2057-2066.

Rainer T. *The new diary: How to use a journal for self guidance and expanded creativity.* Tarcher/Putnam Books, New York, NY. 1978.

Raspe H, Hueppe A, Neuhauser H. Back pain, a communicable disease? *International Journal of Epidemiology.* 2008, 37:69-74.

Rico GL. *Writing the Natural Way: Using Right-Brain Techniques to Release Your Expressive Powers.* J. P. Tarcher, Inc., Los Angeles, CA. 1983.

Roemer L, Litz BT, Orsillo SM, Ehlich PJ, Friedman MJ. Increases in retrospective accounts of war-zone exposure over time: The role of PTSD symptom severity. *Journal of Traumatic Stress.* 1998, 11: 597-605.

Ross JS, Tkach J, Ruggieri PM, Lieber M, Lapresto E. The mind's eye: functional MR imaging evaluation of golf motor imagery. *American Journal of Neuroradiology.* 2003, 24: 1036-44.

Roth G, Assor A, Niemiec CP, Deci EL. The emotional and academic consequences of parental conditional regard. *Developmental Psychology.* 2009, 45: 1119-1142.

Ruden R. *When the Past Is Always Present: Emotional Traumatization, Causes, and Cures.* Taylor and Francis Group, New York, NY. 2011.

Sarno, JE. *The Mindbody Prescription: Healing the body, healing the pain.* Warner Books, New York, NY. 1998.
Sarno JE. *The Divided Mind.* HarperCollins Books, New York, NY. 2006.

Schafe GE, Nader K, Blair HT, LeDoux JE. Memory consolidation of Pavlovian fear conditioning: a cellular and molecular perspective. *Trends in Neurosciences.* 2001, 24: 540-546.

Schmitt DP, Realo A, Voracek M, Allik J. Why can't a man be more like a woman? Sex differences in big five personality traits across 55 cultures. *Journal of Personality and Social Psychology.* 2008, 94:168-182.

Schrader H, Obelieniene D, Bovim G, Surkiene D, Mickeviciene D, Miseviciene I, Sand T. Natural evolution of late whiplash syndrome outside the medicolegal context. *Lancet.* 1996, 347: 1207-11.

Schrader H, Stovner LJ, Obelieniene D, Surkiene D, Mickeviciene D, Bovim G, Sand T. Examination of the diagnostic validity of 'headache attributed to whiplash injury: a controlled, prospective study. *European Journal of Neurology.* 2006, 13: 1226-32.

Schwartz RC, Sweezy M. *Internal Family Systems Therapy.* The Guilford Press, New York. 2020.

Selfridge N, Peterson F. *Freedom from fibromyalgia: The 5-week program proven to conquer pain.* Three Rivers Press, New York, NY. 2001.

Selhub, E, Infusino D. *The Love Response: Your prescription to turn off anger, fear and anxiety.* Ballantine Books, New York, NY. 2009.

Sherman JJ, Turk DC, Okifuji A. Prevalence and impact of posttraumatic stress disorder-like symptoms on patients with fibromyalgia syndrome. *Clinical Journal of Pain.* 2000, 16: 127-134.

Shorter, E. *From paralysis to fatigue: A history of psychosomatic illness in the modern era.* The Free Press, Simon and Schuster, New York, NY. 1992.

Siegel RD. *The mindfulness solution: Everyday practices for everyday problems.* Guilford Press, New York, NY. 2010.

Siegel RD, Urdang MH, Johnson DR. *Back sense: A revolutionary approach to halting the cycle of chronic back pain.* Broadway Books, New York, NY. 2001.

Siegel R, Schubiner H, Schwartz R. Listening to chronic pain: How therapy can heal the hurt. *Psychotherapy Networker,* 2020.

Sifton E. *The Serenity Prayer: Faith and Politics in Times of Peace and War.* W. W. Norton and Company, New York, NY. 2005.

Silverman SM. Opioid induced hyperalgesia: clinical implications for the pain practitioner. *Pain Physician.* 2009, 12: 679-684.

Simotas AC, Shen T. Neck pain in demolition derby drivers. *Archives of Physical Medicine and Rehabilitation.* 2005, 86: 693-6.

Staal JB, deBie RA, deVet HC, Heldebrandt J, Nelemans P. Injection therapy for subacute and chronic low back pain: an updated Cochrane review. *Spine* (Phila PA, 1976). 2009, 34: 49-59.

Stephens R, Atkins J, Kingston A. Swearing as a response to pain. *Neuroreport.* 2009, 20: 1056-1060.

Stephens R, Umland C. Swearing as a response to pain—effect of daily swearing frequency. *The Journal of Pain.* 2011, 12: 1274-1281.

Strine TW, Hootman JM. US national prevalence and correlates of low back and neck pain among adults. *Arthritis Rheumatology.* 2007, 57: 656-65.

Taddio A, Shah V, Gilbert-MacLeod C, Katz J. Conditioning and hyperalgesia in newborns exposed to repeated heel lances. *Journal of the American Medical Association.* 2002, 288: 857-61.

Takamatsu H, Noda A, Murakami Y, Tatsumi M, Ichise R, Nishimura S. A PET study following treatment with a pharmacological stressor, FG7142, in conscious rhesus monkeys. *Brain Research.* 2003, 980: 275-280.

Takatalo J, Karppinen J, Niinimäki J, Taimela S, Näyhä S, Järvelin MR, Kyllönen E, Tervonen O. Prevalence of degenerative imaging findings in lumbar magnetic resonance imaging among young adults. *Spine* (Phila Pa 1976). 2009, 34: 1716-21.

Taub E, Uswatte G, King DK, Morris D, Crago JE, Chatterjee A. A placebo-controlled trial of constraint-induced movement therapy for upper extremity after stroke. *Stroke.* 2006, 37: 1045-1049.

Tolle E. *The Power of Now.* New World Library, Novato, CA and Namaste Publishing, Vancouver, BC. 1999.

Trakhtenberg EC. The effects of guided imagery on the immune system: a critical review. *International Journal of Neuroscience.* 2008, 118: 839-55.

Uomoto JM, Esselman PC. Traumatic brain injury and chronic pain: differential types and rates by head injury severity. *Archives of Physical Medicine and Rehabilitation.* 1993, 74: 61-4.

van der Kolk BA. The body keeps the score: memory and the evolving psychobiology of posttraumatic stress. *Harvard Review of Psychiatry.* 1994, 1: 253-65.

van Houdenhove B, Neerinckx E, Lysens R, Vertommen H, van Houdenhove L, Onghena P, et. al. Victimization in chronic fatigue and fibromyalgia in tertiary care: A controlled study on prevalence and characteristics. *Psychosomatics.* 2001, 42: 21-28.

Vogt BA, Sikes RW. The medial pain system, cingulated cortex, and parallel processing of nociceptive information. *Progress in Brain Research.* 2000, 122: 223-235.

Waber RL, Shiv B, Carmon Z, Ariely D. Commercial features of placebo and therapeutic efficacy. *Journal of the American Medical Association.* 2008, 299: 1016-7.

Wager TD, Rilling JK, Smith EE, Sokolik A, Casey KL, Davidson RJ, Kosslyn SM, Rose RM, Cohen JD. Placebo induced changes in fMRI in the anticipation and experience of pain. *Science.* 2004, 303: 1162-7.

Walitt B, Fitzcharles MA, Hassett AL, Katz RS, Häuser W, Wolfe F. The longitudinal outcome of fibromyalgia: a study of 1555 patients. *Journal of Rheumatology.* 2011, 38: 2238-46.

Wegner, DM. *The Illusion of Conscious Will.* Bradford Books, The Massachusetts Institute of Technology Press, Cambridge, MA. 2002.

Weinstein JN, Tosteson TD, Lurie JD, Tosteson AN, Hanscom B, Skinner JS, Abdu WA, Hilibrand AS, Boden SD, Deyo RA. Surgical vs nonoperative treatment for lumbar disk herniation: the Spine Patient Outcomes Research Trial (SPORT): a randomized trial. *Journal of the American Medical Association.* 2006, 296: 2441-50.

Weinstein JN, Lurie JD, Tosteson TD, Hanscom B, Tosteson AN, Blood EA, Birkmeyer NJ, Hilibrand AS, Herkowitz H, Cammisa FP, Albert TJ, Emery SE, Lenke LG, Abdu WA, Longley M, Errico TJ, Hu SS. Surgical versus nonsurgical treatment for lumbar degenerative spondylolisthesis. *New England Journal of Medicine*. 2007, 356: 2257-70.

Westen D. The scientific status of unconscious processes: Is Freud really dead? *Journal of the American Psychoanalytic Association*. 1999, 47: 1061-1106.

Whalen PJ, Rauch SL, Etcoff NL, McInerney SC, Lee MB, Jenike MA. Masked presentations of emotional facial expressions modulate amygdala activity without explicit knowledge. *Journal of Neuroscience*. 1998, 18: 411-418.

Williams LE, Bargh JA. Experiencing physical warmth promotes interpersonal warmth. *Science*. 2008, 322: 606-607.

Wilson TD. *Strangers to ourselves: Discovering the adaptive unconscious*. The Belknap Press of Harvard University Press, Cambridge, MA. 2002.

Wolfe F. Fibromyalgia wars. *Journal of Rheumatology*. 2009, 36: 671-8.

Yarns BC, Cassidy JT, Jimenez AM. At the intersection of anger, chronic pain, and the brain: A mini-review. *Neuroscience & Biobehavioral Reviews*. 2022, 135: 104558.

Yarns BC, Lumley MA, Cassidy JT, et. al. Emotional Awareness and Expression Therapy Achieves Greater Pain Reduction than Cognitive Behavioral Therapy in Older Adults with Chronic Musculoskeletal Pain: A Preliminary Randomized Comparison Trial. *Pain Medicine* 2020, 21: 2811–2822.

Yunus MB. Fibromyalgia and overlapping disorders: the unifying concept of central sensitivity syndromes. *Seminars in Arthritis and Rheumatism*. 2007, 36: 339-5.

Zafirides P. Existential Psychotherapy: How the search for meaning can heal us. In *The Psychology of Meaning*, edited by Markman KD, Proulx T, Lindberg MJ. American Psychological Association Press, Washington DC. 2013.

index

about the author

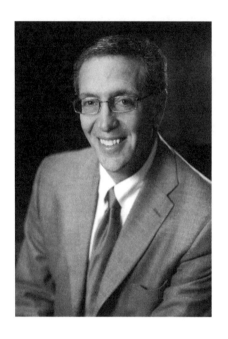

Dr. Howard Schubiner is board certified in pediatrics and internal medicine and is the director of the Mind Body Medicine Center at Ascension Providence Hospital in Southfield, MI. He is a Clinical Professor at Michigan State University College of Human Medicine and is a fellow in the American College of Physicians, and the American Academy of Pediatrics. He has authored more than 100 publications in scientific journals and books and has given more than 500 lectures to scientific audiences regionally, nationally, and internationally. Dr. Schubiner has consulted for the American Medical Association, the National Institute on Drug Abuse, and the National Institute on Mental Health. He is also a senior teacher of mindfulness meditation. He has been included on the list of the Best Doctors in America since 2003. Dr. Schubiner lives in the Detroit area with his wife of thirty-nine years and has two adult children.